A Family
Secret

A Family Secret

The Battersea Tavern Series: Book 2

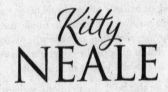

ORION

An Orion paperback
First published in Great Britain in 2022 by Orion Fiction
an imprint of The Orion Publishing Group Ltd
Carmelite House, 50 Victoria Embankment
London EC4Y 0DZ

An Hachette UK Company

3 5 7 9 10 8 6 4 2

A CIP catalogue record for this book is
available from the British Library.

ISBN (Mass Market Paperback) 978 1 4091 9764 5
ISBN (eBook) 978 1 4091 9765 2

Typeset at The Spartan Press Ltd,
Lymington, Hants

Printed and bound in Great Britain by Clays Ltd,
Elcograf S.p.A.

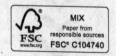

MIX
Paper from
responsible sources
FSC® C104740

www.orionbooks.co.uk

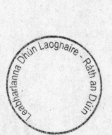

Dedicated to Jay Angel Griffin, an angel on earth and now an angel in heaven. A beautiful soul, gone too soon, remembered with love by all those whose lives you touched xxx

I

7 September 1940
Battersea, London

As Harry Hampton walked through his front door, his heart sank when he was greeted by his wife's sour face and her not-so-dulcet tones.

'Where the bleedin' hell have you been?' Carmen screeched. 'Your lunch is nearly ruined.' Her arms were tightly folded across her chest and her lips were set in a grim line.

Harry removed his trilby hat and placed it on top of the newel post. He was about to explain to Carmen, but before he had a chance to respond, she tutted and answered for him.

'Down the Battersea Tavern again, I suppose. You spend more bloody time in that pub then you do at home. What's the attraction, eh? I know it can't be that Winnie Berry, the fat old cow! So what is it, eh, Harry? Got your eye on her barmaid, have you? You pathetic creature. As if a young woman like Rachel would be interested in an old man like you! Or have you been flashing your cash to try and lure her?'

Harry sighed and rolled his eyes. For Gawd's sake, he thought, the woman knew that he'd been out grafting so there was no need for her to get her knickers in a twist. But of course, Carmen had to get in her little jibe about women and money. He wished that she wouldn't keep mentioning it. And anyway, where he spent his cash was none of her business. But at least his wife didn't suspect that he had feelings for Winnie Berry. His love for Winnie was a well-guarded secret. 'Come on, love, give it a rest, will ya,' he said, feeling exasperated. 'Of course I ain't got my eye on any of the women in the pub. I've only got eyes for you, my sweetness and light,' he placated, hoping against all the odds that she would soften to a bit of his charm.

'Don't give me that, Harry Hampton! You've always had an eye for the ladies, especially the ones who like your money. Well, that Rachel and her bastard baby are welcome to you.'

Harry wished that Carmen wouldn't talk unkindly about Rachel. But, he supposed, his wife was only repeating what a lot of the neighbours were saying. Having a child without a husband meant that Rachel had been labelled a slut. He thought it was a shame, as she seemed like a nice girl. But it was nothing to do with him and he wouldn't dare open his mouth to his wife to defend Rachel. Instead, Harry stepped towards Carmen and wrapped his arms around her slim waist. Her eyes narrowed as she looked at him suspiciously and she kept her arms folded and her back rigid.

'Don't be like that, love. Give your old man a kiss,' Harry teased. He went to place his lips on hers but Carmen quickly turned her face.

'Get orf me, you're drunk. You stink like a brewery and your clothes reek of baccy,' she moaned, stepping back from his clinch.

'I ain't drunk. I've had two pints, that's all.'

'And the rest.'

2

'It's true, sweetheart, honest. I'm not in the pub having a jolly. I'm working. 'Ere you go.' Harry pulled a wad of notes from his trousers pocket and shoved them towards Carmen. 'Not a bad morning's work an' all,' he added proudly.

Carmen didn't hesitate; she grabbed the cash from him and stuffed the money into the pocket of her apron.

'See, you ain't complaining now,' Harry chirped, then mumbled quickly, 'for a change.'

'I heard that! I wouldn't complain if you didn't keep giving me reason to.'

Yeah, you would, Harry thought to himself. His wife was a fine-looking woman but she had a tongue on her that could cut through steel like a hot knife through butter.

Harry shrugged, then sauntered past Carmen as he made his way down the narrow passageway through to the kitchen at the back of the terraced house. His stomach grumbled as he pulled out at a seat at the kitchen table. For all his wife's faults, she always dished up a good meal and Harry was looking forward to his lunch. He was hoping he'd get to eat it in peace but he doubted that would happen as Carmen was clearly in a foul mood.

His wife followed him into the kitchen but he hardly noticed her. He was busy reading the front page of the daily newspaper. It was full of the usual headlines about air battles with the Royal Air Force and the German Luftwaffe and sea clashes.

'See this, love. The RAF are going all out fighting. There's a lot of our blokes getting shot out of the sky. Flamin' Jerries!' Harry said with a shake of his head but his eyes remained fixed on the newspaper.

'I'm sick of hearing about it. If I turn on the wireless,

3

all I hear are news bulletins or first-aid advice. So I'll thank you not to talk about the blasted war over lunch,' Carmen snapped.

Harry wished that he'd kept his mouth shut now. Whenever he opened it, his wife inevitably jumped down his throat. In a bid to change the subject, he asked, 'What's for lunch?'

'Corned-beef hash.'

'Again?' Harry spluttered, instantly regretting his response.

'Yes, again,' Carmen answered tartly. 'I've got two dozen tins stashed under the stairs that you've not flogged yet. If you can't sell it, we may as well eat it. And don't you dare roll your bleedin' eyes at me.'

'I'm sure the corned-beef hash will be smashing,' Harry said, hiding a deep sigh.

Carmen slammed a plate down in front of him and snatched his newspaper away. 'So, let's hear it, then. What fairy tale are you going to tell me this time as your sad excuse for being over an hour late for lunch?'

Harry was about to protest about her pulling away his newspaper but then he thought better of it. He eagerly shoved a forkful of the hash into his mouth and began to chew. All the while, Carmen stared at him accusingly.

'Aren't you having any lunch, love?' he asked.

'I ate an hour ago, at lunchtime,' she replied sarcastically. 'Well? I'm still waiting for an answer about your tardiness.'

'I had to see a man about a dog. I can't sell me stuff if I ain't got nothing to sell.'

'What did you buy?'

'Sausage skins, two dozen chocolate bars and half a dozen bacon joints. I'll get you to cut the bacon up for me and I'll sell it by the slice. It'll go down a treat in the pub.'

'So where is it, then?'

'I'm picking it up tomorrow. And I'll take some of them tins of corned beef out with me tonight and see if I can't shift a few.'

'Yeah, you do that. And while you're at it, you can send our Cheryl home. I don't like her hanging about in the Battersea Tavern. It ain't right for a woman to be in a pub without a man.'

'Come off it, Carmen. There's loads of young women in the pubs nowadays. Let's face it, they're in the factories doing the jobs of men, so why shouldn't they let their hair down?'

'That's just typical of you to stick up for your *little princess*. But I'm telling you, mark my words, no good will come of our daughter drinking in a pub. She'll end up with her reputation in tatters.'

Harry finished his last mouthful of lunch and pushed his plate away. 'That was bloody handsome, that was. Thanks, sweetheart. I tell you what, why don't you come for a drink with me tonight? You'll see for yourself that Cheryl ain't doing no harm.'

'I'll do no such thing!' Carmen answered haughtily. 'You won't get me setting foot in *that place*, thank you very much! And I suggest you put a stop to our Cheryl going in there before she ends up being talked about by the neighbours.'

Harry rolled his eyes again but thankfully Carmen didn't see. She'd taken his plate to the sink and was rinsing it under the tap. From behind, with her raven-black hair pinned high on her head, pert backside and trim hips, Carmen didn't look a day over twenty-five. But time hadn't been so kind to her face and now her olive skin was etched with wrinkles and bags sagged under her dark eyes. Harry still found his wife, at forty-nine years old, to be an attractive woman and he smiled at the memory of when they'd first met. He'd thought she was such an exotic beauty and had assumed she was Spanish. As it turned out, Euphemia, which was her real name, was the product of a one-night stand between her mother and a gypsy boy. When Euphemia had discovered the truth and found out that she'd been born out of wedlock and had a gypsy father, she'd quickly changed her name to Carmen and the Spanish charade had begun. Woe betide Harry if he ever dared to mention his wife's origins. It was a closely guarded secret that even their grown children, Errol and Cheryl, knew nothing about. Yet, regardless of her past, she was quick to hypocritically slate Rachel for being an unmarried mother. But that was typical of his wife; she lacked empathy for anyone.

Carmen turned from the butler sink. 'Are you going to stay for a cuppa?' she asked as she dried her hands on a tea towel. 'The kettle is already on to boil.'

Harry glanced at his watch. It was nearly three o'clock. He'd have to hurry if he wanted to catch his mate, Danny, at the Northcote Road market. 'Sorry, love, I've got to dash. Time is money an' all that.'

He noticed a look of disappointment on Carmen's face and asked, 'Are you all right?'

'Yes, of course I am. Why wouldn't I be?' she spat.

'Excuse me for breathing. I was only asking.'

Carmen's stiff shoulders slumped and she pulled a chair out from the table. She flopped herself down and hung her head. 'I'm bored, Harry. You pop in and out but never stay long and don't get home till late. Cheryl is working long hours at the factory and even today, on a Saturday. And Errol is Lord

6

only knows where. I'm stuck in these four walls day in and day out. I can't even turn on the wireless anymore unless I want to hear about the damned war.'

Harry stared wide-eyed at his wife, somewhat stunned by her revelation. Carmen had always seemed happy enough with her lot and had even boasted about how nice their house was compared to their neighbours, albeit furnished with his ill-gotten gains. It had never occurred to him that she wanted more in her life. 'There's plenty of volunteer things you could get involved with, sweetheart. Old Mrs Hill down the road is collecting woollen jumpers and stuff to make into blankets. Mrs Tinder is organising a gift box scheme for the soldiers overseas and Mrs—'

Carmen interrupted abruptly, 'Yes, thank you, Harry; that will do.'

Oh, of course it will, Harry thought. After all, Carmen wouldn't want to work with any of the women on the street. She didn't get on with most of them but it was her own doing. Over the years, she'd distanced herself from just about all the wives and mothers and those who spoke to her now only did so out of politeness.

Harry scraped his chair back and walked around the table. He placed his arm over his wife's shoulders and lightly kissed her cheek though he had little sympathy for her predicament. 'I'll try and get home a bit earlier tonight and I'll bring you a couple of bottles of stout, eh? Perhaps we can have a game of cards.'

Now it was Carmen who rolled her eyes, very clearly unimpressed.

'I'll see you later, love,' Harry called as he strolled down the passageway.

After grabbing his hat, he closed the front door behind him and immediately his mood felt lighter. His wife was a difficult woman but Harry pushed all thoughts of her to the back of his mind as he began to whistle a happy tune and headed towards the market. It'd be no more shank's pony for him if he managed to catch up with Danny. His mate had a very tidy motorbike and sidecar for sale and Harry was hoping to get it for a good price. Some might call it a luxury but Harry thought it was a necessity. After all, business on the black market was booming. Selling rationed goods and hard-to-come-by items was making Harry a small fortune and the sidecar would be the ideal transport for his stock.

Winnie Berry was pleased to put her feet up after a busy morning as the landlady of the Battersea Tavern. She sat in an armchair next to the hearth in the front room above the pub and kicked off her shoes before giving her aching bunion a gentle rub.

Rachel Robb, her young loyal barmaid and good friend, popped her head around the door. 'Do you want a cuppa, Win?'

'You come and sit yourself down, I'll do it,' Winnie answered and she began to push her plump body out of the chair.

'No, stay where you are,' Rachel protested. 'The kettle is already on.'

Winnie smiled fondly at the girl, grateful for Rachel's caring ways. In fact, since Winnie's husband, Brian, had left almost a year earlier, she was grateful for all the support Rachel had given her. Winnie's mind drifted to Brian. She found herself often thinking about him but not with any fondness. Her husband had been a mean man who'd think nothing of giving her a clout or two. For years, she'd lived under his rule, doing his bidding and never daring to fight back. But everything had changed when Jan came into her life and Winnie had thought that Jan was the child she'd given up for adoption. In order to make things up to her long-lost daughter, Winnie had found an inner strength and had stood up to Brian's tyrannical ways. She wished now that she'd been stronger years earlier and hadn't let Brian ruin her life for so long. *But there's no point crying over spilt milk*, she thought. What's done is done. And though Brian reaped half the profits from the pub, at least they were no longer living under the same roof.

Winnie smiled affectionately at Rachel when the girl returned with two cups of tea. 'I should think Martha will be awake any minute now,' she said as she placed a cup on a table next to Winnie. And right on cue, before Rachel had sat down, they heard Martha crying from the bedroom next door. Winnie chuckled. 'That granddaughter of mine is as regular as clockwork.'

'She really is. She's been asleep for exactly one hour,' Rachel replied as she hurried from the room.

Martha's cries subsided and Rachel returned carrying her baby daughter in her arms, cooing lightly at her.

'Give her here to her nanny,' Winnie said with outstretched arms. 'You drink your tea, love, and I'll have a cuddle.'

Rachel carefully handed Martha to Winnie and threw herself down onto the armchair opposite. 'I'm worn out, Win. She's had me up three times in the night and doesn't sleep past six-thirty in the morning.'

'I know. Babies may be little but they're hard work. Go and have a lie down. I'll keep an eye on Martha.'

'No, but thanks. I wouldn't be able to sleep,' Rachel answered wistfully.

'Are you still worrying about Hilda?'

'Yes. I know it's daft but I can't help thinking that now that Jan has joined the Civil Nursing Reserve, Hilda will get lonely. They spent so much time together making dresses. I'm sure having Jan around helped to keep Hilda sober. And now that Jan has been posted to St Thomas's Hospital, Hilda might go off the rails again.'

'Listen, love. Hilda wasn't a good mother to you. Well, she wasn't any sort of mother at all to you. But you can't fault her as a grandmother to little Martha here. Hilda hasn't touched a drop of booze since she found out that you were pregnant. She made you a promise and she's kept to it. She's trying her best to make up for all the years she lost as your mother.'

'I know, but, like I said, she's always had Jan around and now she hasn't.'

'Time will tell. But there's no point in worrying over something that hasn't happened. 'Ere, I think Martha wants a feed,' Winnie said. She gave her precious granddaughter a gentle kiss on her forehead, savouring the sweet smell of the baby, and then handed her back to Rachel. 'Hilda won't be the only one to miss Jan. I will an' all. She's not my daughter by blood but she is in every other way and I'm ever so proud of her.'

'And so you should be. I'm proud of her too and I'll miss her. Jan's my best friend. It won't be the same here without her.'

'I hope she gets a chance to visit us again soon. It was

lovely to see her last week. I worry myself silly about her so I was glad to hear that the retired nurses are looking after the trainees. Fancy some of them sleeping in the basement of the hospital. Mind you, from what she said, it sounded very comfortable.'

'And didn't she look smashing in her uniform?'

'Oh, she really did! Terry's eyes nearly popped out of his head,' Winnie chortled. 'I'm surprised he hasn't yet asked Jan to marry him. I'd have thought he would have put a ring on her finger, especially as she's going to be working with all those doctors.'

'Terry knows he hasn't got to worry about losing Jan to a doctor. She's smitten with him.'

'They make a lovely couple,' Winnie said, smiling fondly. 'I'll have this cuppa and then I'm going to pop to the post office. I've got another letter to post to her.'

'I can take it, if you like?'

'Thanks, love, but I could do with a bit of fresh air. I was thinking, now that Jan has moved out, we could do with an extra pair of hands, so I reckon it'll be a good idea to rent out her room to someone who can work behind the bar with me.'

'But I can manage with Martha and working downstairs.'

'I know you can, love, but as she grows, she'll demand more attention. Anyway, I could do with the extra money coming in. What with Brian demanding half the profits and then there's the increased taxes on the beer, a couple of bob a week from renting that room will come in handy.'

'It ain't right that Mr Berry takes money for doing nothing.'

Winnie sighed. 'You can say that again. He does bugger

all but at least I get to have my name above the door so he can't walk back in here and throw me out.'

'I suppose, but it still doesn't seem right.'

'It ain't,' Winnie said through tight lips. 'My old man's a sly sod! He realised he wouldn't be able to sell the place for what it's worth, not with a war on. And he's not prepared to work in the pub himself. So here's me, putting in all the hours while he's sitting pretty. But what could I do? He had me over a barrel. It was either agree to his demands or risk him taking the pub off me. But it's me having the last laugh. Between you and me, I'm making a bit more money than I'm putting though the books.'

Rachel looked at Winnie with her eyes stretched wide. 'How?' she asked, sounding surprised.

'I've been buying the spirits from Have-it Harry and now he's confident he can get his hands on some beer an' all.'

'Isn't that illegal?'

'Shush, yes, of course it is. Everything Harry sells is on the black market and mostly through the back door. You know me, I'm as straight as a die usually but needs must.'

'I can't say I blame you, Win. And Harry makes a lot of people's lives a bit easier.'

'Yes, for those who can afford to buy from him. He ain't cheap. But a lot of folk like to top up their rations.'

'He does good trade in the pub.'

'He does and I get a discount for allowing him to work out of my pub, so it's a win-win situation for us both.' Winnie hoped she wasn't blushing as she spoke about Harry. Even the mention of his name gave her butterflies and left her feeling flushed.

Rachel yawned and then asked, 'Have you got anyone in mind for Jan's old room?'

Martha had fallen asleep on Rachel's breast and Winnie could see that Rachel's eyes were looking heavy. 'Yes, love; Lucy Little from the florist's. She was telling me that the flowers make her sneeze, she can't stand it. But she can't afford to leave the job because she'd lose her room, which comes with it.'

'I don't think I've ever said more than two words to her but she seems nice enough,' Rachel replied before yawning again.

'Right, that's it. You can hardly keep your eyes open. Go on, off to bed, the pair of you. And don't worry about Hilda. She won't let you or Martha down, I'm sure of it.'

'Thanks, Win. I think I will have a nap but don't let me sleep for too long. Give me a shout when you get back from the post office.'

'Will do, love,' Winnie replied as Rachel slumped off.

Winnie checked the clock on the mantelpiece and saw it was just after four o'clock. She squeezed her aching feet back into her shoes and winced as she heaved herself out of the green, wing-backed armchair. After wrapping a scarf over her head and tying it under her chin, she pulled on her coat, grabbed her handbag and went downstairs. She trudged towards the local shops in the hope of seeing Lucy Little. Now that Winnie knew that Rachel wasn't adverse to the idea of Lucy living with them, she could put the offer to the young lady and she felt confident that Lucy would readily accept. But first things first – Winnie's priority was to post her letter to dear Jan.

★

It had taken Winnie a while to walk to the shops and she'd had a good natter with Mrs Dawes, the wife of the post-master. Winnie had felt fit to burst with pride as she'd told the woman all about Jan working at St Thomas's Hospital in Westminster. It sounded very well-to-do! And now, as she made her way to the florist's, Winnie was filled with a warm feeling, knowing that Jan would soon receive the letter. She'd written about the local gossip from the pub and told her that Rachel and Terry both sent their love. She pictured Jan reading the letter with a smile on her face.

Just as Winnie arrived at the florist's, Lucy was coming out of the shop, her eyes red-rimmed and watering.

'Hello, love, are you all right?' Winnie asked, concerned.

'Hello, Mrs Berry. Oh, this,' Lucy said, indicating her eyes. 'Yes, I'm fine, thanks. It's the flowers that make me like this. I was just about to lock up. Did you want to buy anything?'

'No, but I was hoping to catch you. I've got a proposition for you.'

Lucy sniffed and pulled a handkerchief from her coat pocket, then blew her nose. 'Sorry, what is it?'

'Well, I thought you might like to come and work in the pub and rent a room upstairs. You'd be living with me, Rachel and baby Martha,' Winnie replied with a broad smile.

'Oh,' Lucy mumbled before lowering her eyes to the ground.

Winnie had been expecting Lucy to jump at her offer and wondered why the girl didn't seem to be very keen. 'Is something wrong?' she asked.

'Erm, no, it's – erm – ever so kind of you.'

'So what's the problem?'

'I don't know how to put this, but – but it's Rachel and the baby.'

'What about them?'

'She's ... well, Rachel's not married. I'm not sure that it would be a good idea for me to be living with her, you know, in case I get tarred with the same brush.'

Winnie sucked in a sharp lungful of air and her chin jutted forward. 'How dare you insinuate that Rachel is anything but a nice, decent girl! And that baby is *my* granddaughter!'

Lucy hung her head. 'I'm sorry, Mrs Berry, I didn't mean to offend you.'

'Too late, young lady; you have and you can stick my offer where the sun don't shine!' Winnie snapped. She was about to spin on her heel and march off when the unmistakable sound of the air-raid warning siren suddenly filled the air.

Lucy looked at Winnie, her sore eyes now filled with fear. She gasped and cried out, 'Oh, no! The Jerries are coming! I knew they would! They're gonna kill us all!'

'It's all right. It'll likely be a false alarm again. But get yourself off to the public shelter, better to be safe than sorry.'

Lucy began gasping for breath and her face drained of all colour.

'Did you hear me? You need to get to a shelter,' Winnie repeated.

The girl stared blankly ahead, her breaths rapid. Winnie took Lucy squarely by the shoulders and gave her a gentle shake. 'Go to a shelter, Lucy,' she repeated firmly.

Lucy nodded but remained rooted to the spot. All around, people were running, some were crying. The sound of the sirens screeched loudly. Winnie could feel the panic in the air. 'Come on,' she said impatiently, grabbing Lucy's arm, dragging her along the street. She didn't have time for this. She had to get back to the pub. To Rachel and Martha. But she couldn't leave Lucy in the street, paralysed with fear.

As they neared the public air-raid shelter, Winnie was relieved to see one of her customers. ' 'Ere, Phil, take Lucy with you,' she said, gently pushing the girl towards the middle-aged man.

'Ain't you coming in?' he asked.

'No, Rachel's all alone at the pub.'

'You won't get back there in time. Come in here, it'll be safer.'

Winnie didn't reply. She was already hurrying in the op-posite direction and back towards the Battersea Tavern. Her legs wouldn't move fast enough and she was beginning to struggle for breath. She heard the sound of an engine beside her and looked over to see Have-it Harry Hampton riding a motorbike with a sidecar.

He pulled up against the kerb and shouted, 'Get in,' nod-ding towards the small carriage.

'I ain't getting in that contraption!'

'It'll get you back to the pub at double speed. Just get in, woman.'

Winnie huffed but she knew that Harry was right. She would get back to Rachel a lot quicker in the sidecar than she would on foot. Reluctantly, she climbed in though it was a struggle. Harry sped off and soon they arrived outside the pub. He was quick to jump off the bike and rushed to help pull her out of the carriage.

As she clambered out, Winnie looked skyward, horrified to see hundreds of planes overhead. 'Good grief!' she muttered and swallowed hard.

Harry looked up too. 'Christ alive, there's bloody loads of 'em! Are you all right? I need to get back to Carmen.'

'Yes, yes, Harry. Go. Thanks for the lift,' she answered hastily.

Winnie fumbled in her handbag for the back-door key. The thud of the ack-ack guns and the hammering sound of gunfire overhead made her heart race. She panicked. Finally, finding the key, she let herself in to see Rachel sitting on the stairs with Martha screaming in her arms.

'I'm scared, Win. What do I do? I have to protect my baby!'

'It's all right, love,' Winnie soothed, though she was scared too. She'd never seen so many Luftwaffe planes in the sky before and had a terrible feeling that something awful was about to be unleashed on London. There was no time left to get to the public shelter on the adjoining street. 'Down to the cellar, quickly,' she said and beckoned Rachel towards the door.

'But what if the pub gets bombed? The whole thing will come down on top of us.'

'We won't get bombed, just try and keep calm.'

They hurried down the stairs to the cellar and Winnie took Martha as Rachel pulled an old bar stool from against the wall. Instantly, Martha stopped crying when Winnie held her against her ample chest.

'Sit down, Win.'

'No, I'm fine. I'll sit just here.' She passed the baby back to Rachel and then sat on the third step of the stairs.

'Oh, Win, I'm so scared.'

'Shush now, let me listen. Just sit tight. It'll be all right. I think the planes are passing over us.'

'Are you sure? I think I can hear explosions,' Rachel cried, tears rolling down her cheeks.

'They're a long way off. Probably the other side of the river,' Winnie answered, suddenly worried for Jan's safety.

Everyone had been dreading this. Customers had talked about the Germans invading by air but Winnie had never really believed it would happen. Granted, the aerodromes had been attacked but she'd been sure that the Royal Air Force would have held off the Germans from bombing London. She shook her head in disbelief, still reeling at the sheer amount of planes she'd seen in the sky.

'What, Win? What are you thinking?' Rachel asked.

'Nothing, love,' Winnie lied. She couldn't tell Rachel what she'd seen flying over their heads. The girl was already in a bad enough state. 'I was just thinking that Jan is probably going to be busy. It's not a nice thought.'

'I can't bear it! It's too awful to contemplate.'

They sat in silence, both tense and listening for every muffled sound. The planes' engines became a distant hum and eventually the aerial gunfire ceased. The air-raid warning siren wailed out to signal the all-clear. At last, after a tense hour or two, Winnie let out a long sigh of relief. They'd come through it unscathed though she knew that tomorrow's papers would be filled with tragic news of Londoners being killed by German explosives.

Winnie's mind turned. If only she could speak to Jan. She needed to know about the welfare of her unofficially adopted daughter. *Please be safe, Jan*, she prayed in her head. *Please, God, keep my Jan safe.*

2

Cheryl Hampton rushed through the front door and dashed into the living room, desperate to know that her family were safe and accounted for. She barged into the room to find her mother having a go at her father, as usual.

Her mother was seething and speaking to her dad through gritted teeth. 'I don't give two monkeys where you shift the stuff to; just get it out of our bleedin' shelter.'

Her father looked exasperated as he replied, 'I ain't got nowhere else to stash it right now, Carmen. Be reasonable, eh, sweetheart?'

Cheryl panted for breath as she looked resentfully from her mother to her father. 'Hello. Yes, I'm fine, thanks for asking,' she spat sarcastically.

Her mother glanced across and eyed Cheryl up and down as she said, 'I can see for myself that you're fine, I don't need to ask you.'

Her father at least offered some sympathy. 'Sorry, darlin'. That was a bit of a scare for us all, weren't it? Did you take cover in the factory shelter?'

'Yeah,' Cheryl answered and gulped. 'It was horrible. We

were packed in like sardines. There was nowhere to sit and no toilets or anything.'

'At least you had a shelter you could get into. Our Anderson is filled to the rafters with your father's pinched stuff. It's nice to know that he's more worried about his *junk* getting blown to smithereens than he is about his wife and kids!'

'Give it a rest, Carmen. It ain't like that and you know it. How was I supposed to know that the Jerries would come? We ain't needed that shelter since I dug it in so I thought I might as well put it to good use. And it ain't junk. That's our rent money in there and more besides.'

Cheryl had heard enough. Her parents were always arguing over something petty. She stamped out of the room and up the stairs to her bedroom. Their voices drifted up behind her. Her mother's shrill nagging and her father's pandering, trying to make a joke out of everything. Cheryl slammed her door shut to block out their noise. It hadn't seemed to bother either of them that at least a few hundred enemy planes had been directly above their heads. They didn't appear to be aware that bombs had exploded just the other side of the Thames and probably some in Battersea too. People were dead. Buildings were on fire. Cheryl had seen the smoke billowing into the sky and gloomily hanging over the city. What if the bombs had landed on their house? She shuddered at the thought.

Cheryl plonked herself down onto the edge of her bed and held her hands out in front of her. They were still shaking. She'd put on a brave face in the shelter but if the truth be known, she'd been terrified. Her best friend, Yvonne, had held her hand and squeezed so tightly that it had hurt Cheryl and numbed her fingers. But she hadn't complained and instead had tried to offer Yvonne some comforting reassurance. When the all-clear had sounded and they'd emerged from the shelter, Yvonne's mother had run towards them and thrown her arms around Yvonne, who appeared to be equally pleased to see her mum. It had been touching to watch. Cheryl's mother never offered any displays of affection. In fact, the woman barely had a kind word to say. She wished her mother were more like Yvonne's mum.

The bedroom door flew open, making Cheryl jump and snapping her from her thoughts. She looked up to see her big brother, Errol, filling the door frame. He was easily a foot taller than her petite height of five feet.

'You all right, Sis?' he asked.

'Yes, I'm fine, thanks. Are they still arguing downstairs?'

'No. Dad's out the back emptying the shelter. Mum's making tea. What were they rowing about this time?'

'Dad's stuff in the shelter. Mum couldn't get in when Moaning Minnie went off.'

'Oh, right, yeah, that would do it,' Errol said and chuckled. 'I'm going out again. I just wanted to check on you.'

'Thanks. It's nice to know that someone cares.' Cheryl smiled affectionately at her brother. She thought he looked very smart in his made-to-measure suit and long wool coat. Not like the other lads in Battersea who dressed in donkey jackets and flat caps. Errol gave her a wink and then sauntered off, smoothing his dark hair with his hand. She smiled to herself, thinking about how Yvonne had had a crush on him for years. But Yvonne wasn't Errol's type of girl. She was far too plain, sweet and well behaved for him. Errol liked to maintain his reputation as a bad boy and always had a woman on his arm who matched his style. But the women came and went. They never lasted long and Cheryl was glad of that. She didn't think that any of her brother's girlfriends had been good enough for him. Especially his latest ex, Stephanie Reynolds. Cheryl had been happy to see the back of that one!

Carmen called up the stairs. 'Are you coming down for your dinner?'

London was burning. People were dying. The last thing Cheryl wanted was food. 'No,' she yelled back.

'It wasn't a request, young lady. Get your ungrateful backside down here. I'm not wasting good food.'

Cheryl drew in a long breath and sighed heavily. There was no point in trying to argue with her mother. She stood up and then realised that she was still wearing her hat and coat, so she removed them quickly before traipsing down the stairs and into the kitchen.

Her father came through the back door and washed his hands at the sink as her mother banged down three plates on the table. Errol rarely ate with them. In fact, their mother didn't bother to cook for him anymore. Cheryl missed him being around. She missed his banter and his cheeky grin. He still lived at home with them but spent most of his time with his mates.

Cheryl's father caught her attention by waving his fork at her. 'I'm off out down the pub after tea but I want you to stay at home tonight and keep your mother company.'

'But—'

'No buts,' he interrupted. 'You're to stay indoors tonight. End of conversation.'

It wasn't like her father to be so firm and though normally she could wrap him around her little finger, she shrugged and reluctantly agreed. But the thought of spending the evening with her mother wasn't at all appealing. Neither was the thought of having fun in the pub when London had been attacked by German bombers. And to make matters worse, Cheryl feared that the planes would soon return.

Once the all-clear had sounded, Winnie had opened the pub. As expected, her worried customers had soon begun to stream through the door, either eager to hear of any news or wanting a stiff drink. She'd heard that several bombs had dropped on Clapham, only a few miles up the road. And one in Chelsea. There was a rumour that two had landed in Battersea but no one could say where. It was too scarily close! She'd had no word from Jan but guessed that the girl would be run ragged caring for the injured who would have been brought into the hospital. Her Jan, a nurse, *fancy that*, Winnie thought, honoured but worried sick to the pit of her stomach.

The door opened again and when Winnie saw Lucy Little walk in, she glared angrily at the girl. Lucy had some audacity coming here after the derogatory comment she'd made about Rachel earlier. 'Yes, what do you want?' Winnie asked, her tone unfriendly.

'I've come to thank you for getting me to the shelter,' Lucy answered sheepishly.

'Right. You've thanked me. Now you can bugger off.'

'I – erm – wanted to apologise too. I shouldn't have said what I said.'

'No, you shouldn't have.'

'I was wondering if your generous offer still stands?'

Winnie was about to bark at the girl that no, the offer most definitely did not stand, but she glanced up and down the bar.

Three customers were already waiting for refills and another two had just walked in. Rachel was busy upstairs feeding Martha. Winnie needed help and she needed it immediately. 'I suppose so. But any scathing remarks and you'll be out on your ear.'

'Thanks, Mrs Berry. I'll go and collect my things.'

'No, that can wait. I need you behind the bar.'

Lucy nodded but looked pensive.

'Don't worry, my customers don't bite. Throw your coat over the bannisters out the back. Then get behind the bar and smile. You'll soon get the hang of it.'

Winnie showed Lucy how to pull a pint and how to operate the cash register. The girl was a quick learner and had a good way with the customers. Winnie found herself beginning to warm to her.

Moments later, the door opened again and Winnie's stomach flipped at the sight of Harry. He sauntered in, looking as confident as always and twice as smart. 'Here's Have-it Harry,' she said and then instructed Lucy, 'Get him a bottle of light ready.'

Harry Hampton stopped to have a chat at every table between the entrance and the bar.

'Why do you call him *Have-it* Harry?' Lucy asked.

Winnie grinned. 'Because whatever it is you need, Harry will have it.'

'Oh, I see. Do you think he will have any stockings?'

'I know he has.'

'Would you mind asking for me please, Mrs Berry?'

'Don't be shy, you can ask him yourself. 'Ere, Harry, Lucy would like a word,' Winnie called across the smoky room.

Considering the air raid a couple of hours earlier, Winnie

thought there was a good atmosphere in the pub. She was about to ask Piano Pete to play a few tunes on the piano but her heart sank quickly when she heard the familiar wailing of the siren once more.

'Oh no,' Lucy cried, 'they're coming back!'

'Right, that's your lot, folks. Come on, off you go, as fast as you can, please,' Winnie ordered. She came around from the bar to usher her customers out of the door. 'Look after yourselves,' she reminded them as they left.

'I'll see you tomorrow, Winnie,' Harry said hastily as he dashed out.

Once the pub was empty, Winnie locked the door and turned around to see Rachel looking frightened, standing next to an equally scared-looking Lucy. 'It's all right. We'll be fine. Rachel, you know what to do. Take Lucy downstairs with you. I'll fetch a few things and will be down shortly. Go on now, don't just stand there gawping at me.'

'This way,' Rachel said to Lucy and she led her towards the cellar.

Winnie shook her head. This was no way for Martha to be brought up. The poor baby screamed every time the sirens sounded and Rachel shouldn't have to be worried for her baby's life. It wasn't fair. None of it was fair. *Bloody Germans*, she thought. *Bloody stupid German men! It's always men. They're more trouble than they're worth.* Her husband, Brian, had been a useless article and nasty with it. And her son, David, hadn't been any better. She'd never admit it to anyone but she thought about David every day. She wondered where he was living and what he was doing. Was he happy? He didn't deserve to be after what he'd done to Rachel – taking advantage of her when she'd been too drunk to object and abandoning her with an unborn child. Not that Rachel wanted anything to do with him. The only good thing to come out of the sorry mess was Martha. And she was such a bonny baby. The apple of Winnie's eye. But what an awful world for the poor child to have been brought into – a world where men killed other men by the hundreds and thousands; where bombs dropped on the heads of innocent women and children; and where a good, kind mother was ostracised for having a baby without a husband. Winnie was under no illusion that poor Martha would grow up having names and abuse thrown at her. People could be so cruel.

The lights suddenly went out, throwing the pub into darkness and making Winnie gasp. She felt under the bar for the candles and a box of matches. This was all she needed! After lighting a candle, she hurried to the small back kitchen. There, she grabbed a loaf of bread, a plate of leftover meat, a jar of pickled onions and the biscuit tin. She stuffed it all into a shopping basket and made her way back through the pub to the cellar, picking up three bottles of ginger beer on route.

'Mind yourself on the stairs, Win,' Rachel called up. 'I think we've had a power cut.'

'Yes, love, I know. It's fine, I've got a candle,' Winnie answered as she precariously walked down the steps. She was always careful on the steps now; she'd fallen down them just before Christmas last year and had badly twisted her ankle.

Lucy rushed towards her and relieved her of the shopping bag.

Thankfully, Martha had quietened down and had fallen asleep. But even deep in the cellar, they could hear the muted sounds of the battling planes overhead.

'Anyone fancy a bite to eat?' Winnie asked, trying to sound jolly.

'How can you think about food at a time like this?' Rachel cried.

'I've got a feeling we're going to be down here for a while and a lot more often, so we might as well get used to it. Once this raid is over, I'll make it more comfortable. We could do with some blankets and pillows. And maybe that old deckchair that's under the stairs. I'll clear that shelf and stock it with a few provisions. Don't you worry, girls, this cellar will be like a home from home by the time I've finished with it.'

'Oh, Win, I know you're trying to keep our spirits up but I can't stand the thought of me and Martha being holed up down here.'

'It's either this or the public shelter. We need to make the best of it.'

Rachel sighed. 'You're right. I'm just so scared.'

'I know, love. We all are. But we've got to believe that we'll be all right. Now, who wants a cold-chicken sandwich and a pickle?'

Rachel turned her nose up but Lucy was quick to say, 'Yes, please.'

Winnie had forgotten the butter and any utensils and plates. She made a mental note of what to bring down to the cellar for future use – including candles and matches. As she pulled the bread apart, she noticed her hands were trembling. This wouldn't do. She couldn't allow Rachel and Lucy to see that she was just as scared as they were. *Pull yourself together*, she firmly told herself. *You're the head of this household!*

Winnie handed Lucy the sandwich with steadier hands.

'Thank you, Mrs Berry,' the girl said softly.

'Call me Winnie. There's a few house rules that we may as well discuss now. I won't allow any overnight visitors and no men are permitted upstairs without prior consent from me.'

Lucy nodded as she chewed the bread and chicken.

'I'll deduct the rent for your room directly from your wages along with the cost of food and bills. You can use the living room and kitchen whenever you like. We normally eat our meals together. You're more than welcome to join us. Clean up after yourself. Be considerate to others. And that's about it.'

'Sounds good to me. I'm looking forward to having some company. I was a bit lonely in my old room. I never saw the other people in the house.'

'Ain't you got any family?' Winnie probed.

'Yeah. My mum lives near the Latchmere. I pop in once a week but I don't stay long because I can't stand her husband and he doesn't like me either. Two of my older brothers are off fighting. One's in France; the other is on a ship somewhere. And I've got three sisters all younger than me. My mum's got her hands full with them.'

'Why don't you like your mum's husband?' Rachel asked.

'He's horrible. He's taken the strap to me for no reason!'

'Oh, that's awful. He doesn't sound like a nice man.'

'He isn't. My real dad died when I was seven. Then Mum married Sydney and had my sisters. He never hits them. It was only ever me who got it. I couldn't wait to move out.'

Winnie made herself as comfortable as she could on the stairs and listened to the young ladies having a natter. She thought it was nice for Rachel to have a girl around of her own age, especially now that Jan had moved out. Their conversation changed to music. They seemed to be getting on well and had a lot in common. Both were slim and blonde, and Winnie thought they could easily be mistaken for sisters.

She must have nodded off as she was woken by the sound of Martha's cries.

'Sorry, Win, I tried to keep her quiet,' Rachel said as she put the baby to her breast.

Winnie wasn't sure how long she'd been asleep for but her neck ached and the candle had burned right down. 'What's the time?' she mumbled and strained her eyes to look at her watch. She couldn't believe what she was seeing and blinked hard and looked again. 'It's nearly half past four in the morning. Haven't them bleedin' Germans got beds to go to?'

Rachel chuckled and Lucy joined in.

'What? What's so funny?' Winnie asked.

'You've a way with words,' Rachel answered.

'Well, this is silly. They're taking liberties. People have got jobs to get up for and could do without all this flippin' racket and malarkey.'

'I don't think the Germans are worried about Londoners not getting a good night's sleep.'

'No, I don't suppose they are, the inconsiderate sods,' Winnie said with a sigh and she tutted.

Moments later, Martha began to cry again as the sirens sounded the all-clear.

'Huh, about time too,' Winnie said, pushing herself to her feet. Her body felt stiff and she ached from the cold and damp step. 'Right, let's have a cuppa and then get straight to bed. Rachel can lend you a nightie, Lucy, and you can collect your things from your old place tomorrow.'

'I hope you don't mind being bossed around,' Rachel whispered to Lucy, 'Because you'd better get used to it.'

'Oi,' Winnie quipped jovially, 'it's rude to whisper.'

'I think I'm going to really enjoy living here,' Lucy said and she smiled.

Good, thought Winnie. She'd had her reservations about Lucy at first but after seeing how well she and Rachel had rubbed along together, Winnie believed Lucy was going to become a very welcome part of their family. And as Winnie had discovered, family didn't have to mean that you shared the same blood.

3

'I hope we don't have to spend too many nights in that shelter,' Carmen moaned as she placed a plate of toast on the kitchen table.

Harry yawned and helped himself to two slices. He, too, hoped that the night raids wouldn't become a regular occurrence. He'd never admit it to his wife but he'd been terrified. And though the shelter offered some protection, he knew they wouldn't stand a chance of surviving a direct hit from a bomb. He'd been so relieved when they'd heard the all-clear and right now, even with Carmen's whinging, he'd never been so pleased to be in his own kitchen. It had been awfully cramped in the Anderson. The smell of damp soil had bothered him all night and the small dug-out had lacked any comfort. As he lathered butter thickly onto the toast, his mind turned with ideas of how he could add a bit of luxury to the place.

'Harry!' Carmen barked. 'That butter has to last us all week. It's rationed.'

'Yeah, yeah, I know. Don't worry, I'll get you some more.'

'You'd better. And you can get me some eggs too.'

Harry nodded but he was deep in thought about army camp beds and gas lights.

Cheryl came into the kitchen and greeted them sleepily. 'Morning. Cor, what a night that was! I hope that's the last we see of those bombers.'

Harry glanced at his daughter. She looked tired. Dark circles ringed her eyes and her cheeks lacked their usual rosiness. With her black hair, just like her mother's, she looked ghostly. 'Are you all right, sweetheart?' he asked.

'Yes, Dad, just knackered. I'm just glad it's a Sunday and I haven't got to go to work today.'

'Don't you worry, my girl. We won't have another miserable night like last night. I'll soon have that shelter looking and feeling like Buckingham Palace.'

'Ha ha, thanks, Dad. But I suppose we shouldn't complain. At least we've still got a house. Didn't Errol come home?'

'No,' Carmen snapped. 'It wouldn't occur to your brother to let us know if he's alive or not. Never mind that I'm worried sick about him. He's selfish to the core.'

'Aw, Mum, I'm sure he'll be home soon. He'll be tired like the rest of us and probably fell asleep after the air raid.'

'You would stick up for him, wouldn't you?'

'What's that supposed to mean?'

'You and your brother, as thick as thieves. I've heard you both talking about me behind my back.'

'No, we don't.'

'Don't lie to me, Cheryl. And neither one of you is the least bit grateful for the meals I dish up or the clean sheets on your beds every week. I'm just a bloody skivvy to you both.'

'No, Mum, of course we're grateful.'

32

'I never hear either one of you offering to cook the dinner or do the laundry. And Errol treats this place like a hotel!'

Harry sucked in a deep breath before slamming his hand down hard on the table. 'That's enough!' he yelled. 'For once, I'd like to eat my breakfast in peace.'

Cheryl stared at him, her mouth gaping and her eyebrows raised. Carmen glared at him with narrowed eyes.

'Thank you,' he said, enjoying the sudden silence, though he knew it wouldn't last long.

'I'm going back to bed,' Cheryl stated sulkily. She scraped her chair back before throwing Harry a look of disdain, then stamped out of the room. Harry grinned inwardly. His daughter was spoiled and he knew it was his fault. She wasn't used to him raising his voice at her and now would probably sulk until tomorrow.

Once the door had slammed behind his daughter, Carmen hissed, 'Don't ever shout at me again in my own kitchen.'

Harry threw his piece of toast down onto his plate and rose to his feet. He'd had enough of Carmen telling him what he could and couldn't do. 'It's my house, woman. I'll raise my voice wherever and whenever I like,' he growled.

'Oh, will you, indeed? In that case, you can sleep on the sofa from now on and cook your own flamin' meals and clean your own rotten house. How would you like that, eh?'

Harry sighed. He was never going to win. 'All right, all right, you've made your point,' he answered and smiled at his wife though his smile didn't reach his eyes. 'I'll see you later,' he added, before giving Carmen a light peck on the cheek.

Outside, Harry threw his trilby into the sidecar and pulled his peaked-cap crash helmet on, aware of the smell of burning hanging in the air over London. The sun hadn't quite risen over the rooftops but he could see an unusual orange glow in the distance.

'That's fires burning. Poor beggars have taken a right battering over there,' Mr Turnbull said.

Harry glanced over his shoulder at his elderly next door neighbour and nodded his head.

The old man curled his lip in disgust. 'The first lot of bombs caused the fires. When the Jerries came over the second time, the fires led 'em straight to London. They just followed the flames. Bloody clever, the crafty gits.' Mr Turnbull pulled his collar up and his flat cap down. 'I'll be seeing, you, Harry. Keep your family safe, man.'

'Yeah, thanks, will do.' Harry threw his leg over the motorbike and looked again towards the orange glow from East London. The Luftwaffe had sustained their attack right into the early hours of the morning. The damage would be substantial. Harry dreaded to think about it and quickly pushed the thoughts from his head. He turned the key in his bike and kick-started the engine, satisfied with the sound of the roar from the motor. Carmen had moaned about the noise. She'd said that all the neighbours' net curtains would be twitching and the bike would wake the dead. But Carmen moaned about everything.

Harry sped along the main street. The shops wouldn't be open today but there were plenty of people going about their business. He guessed that the atmosphere would be subdued and that most folk would be exhausted after the all-night attack. But there was still business to be done and money to be made. And Harry had a deal in the pipeline that was going to make him a very tidy profit.

He pulled up at Walter Griffin's garage, pleased to see the

wooden door was already open. But as he removed his crash helmet, he was surprised to see Errol inside, talking with Walter. 'Wotcha, Son,' he called.

Errol turned and looked surprised. He mumbled something to Walter and then walked towards Harry looking somewhat guilty.

'What are you doing here?' Harry asked, suspiciously.

'Having a chat with Walter. It ain't against the law, is it?'

'Don't get clever with me, Son. What are you talking to Walter about?'

'This and that.'

'And what exactly is *this and that*?'

'Nothing.'

'Well, you can talk about *nothing* later. You need to get yourself home now. Your mother is worried about you.'

'Give us a lift?'

'No, I need to have a word with Walter. I'll see you down the Battersea Tavern at lunchtime for a drink?'

Errol shrugged his broad shoulders. 'Yeah, all right,' he answered dully before sloping away.

Harry placed his helmet on the sidecar and walked up to Walter with his hand extended. 'Hello, mate. How are you diddling? I hope my boy weren't being a bother.'

Walter ran his hands through his greased-back brown hair and then shook Harry's hand but he looked awkward and avoided meeting Harry's eyes. 'Hello, Harry. I'm – erm – a bit busy right now.'

Harry wanted to wipe his hand on something and looked around the garage for a cloth or rag. 'It's all right, I won't keep you. I just wanted to sort out the details about the ration books. Cash on delivery. I'll have the whole lot. Twenty books, you said. Can you have them ready for tomorrow?'

'Yeah, about that, Harry. The thing is, I've already sold them, mate. To your Errol, in fact, and he paid a good price an' all.'

Harry's head snapped round to glare at his so-called friend. 'You what? But we had a deal,' he blurted incredulously.

'Yeah, I know, but all is fair in love and war. Sorry, but Errol offered me a few bob more than you was willing to pay. What's a bloke to do, eh?'

Harry was fuming. He'd known Walter for over forty years, since they'd been at school together. 'Huh, thanks, *mate*. Thanks a bleedin' lot!'

'Don't be like that. You can't tell me that you wouldn't have done the same.'

'No, Walter, I wouldn't have. I've got a thing called *loyalty* towards my friends. If you don't know what it means, look it up in the dictionary!'

Harry stormed out of the garage and climbed back onto his bike. He couldn't believe he'd been stitched up by his oldest friend and his own son. Well, he wouldn't stand for it. Errol would have to hand over the ration books and Harry would give him the price he was going to pay to Walter. Errol would be out of pocket but that would teach his son a lesson.

He raced off in pursuit of Errol, keen to get his hands on the books before his son sold any of them. Harry needed them. He had people waiting for their *extra* books. He had orders to fulfil and a reputation to maintain. They didn't call him Have-it Harry for nothing and he wasn't about to start letting people down.

★

Winnie was on tenterhooks worrying about Jan, though she tried her utmost to put on a cheery smile for her customers. 'There you go, Len,' she said and placed his usual bottle of stout on the bar before passing him his pewter tankard. 'Did you manage to get much sleep last night?' she asked the old man.

'Not a lot. Me and Renee got under the kitchen table. It was better than nothing but it weren't much fun trying to get up off the floor this morning, not with our old bones. We'll probably have another night of it. I wouldn't be surprised if they come back again later.'

'Oh, Len, I really hope not!'

Len didn't normally speak much and mostly sat quietly supping his stout. But he had plenty to say about the Germans and continued, 'Seems to me that the Hun have changed tactics. They ain't aiming for our airfields no more. That was a deliberate attack on London. I heard that there's planes down over Maidstone and Deal, but I dunno if they're ours or not. If it were the Hun, it won't stop 'em from returning.'

'I've never seen so many planes in the sky,' Winnie replied with a shudder as she recalled the shocking sight. She thought it was strange that, in an eerie sort of way, the early evening sunlight glistening on the planes had made them look almost beautiful.

Bernie walked in next and tipped his flat cap at Winnie. He was a man of short stature but packed with energy. Just watching him wore Winnie out. He always seemed to be darting about like a blue-arsed fly.

'Just a quick brandy, Win. My nerves are shot to pieces,' Bernie said and he placed a few coins on the counter. 'I've only popped in to see Have-it. Is he about?'

'Not yet but I'm sure he'll be here soon. Are you all right?'

'Yeah, I am, but my brother and sister-in-law have just turned up at my house. They're from over Shoreditch way. The poor buggers got bombed out last night. They said there was an almighty bang that shook the shelter in their backyard. Dirt and mud came in through the joints. They thought they were gonna get buried alive! Then to top it all, when they came out of the shelter this morning, their house was as flat as a pancake.'

'Oh no, that's terrible!'

'I know. It could have been us. Battersea got off light on all accounts. Me sister-in-law said the fires over her way were burning out of control. They were all joining up into one big inferno. She said there was hundreds of fire engines; they came from outside of London too. But she reckons everyone over the East End is in good spirits, despite the dead and injured. They salvaged what they could from the house and cadged a lift over to us.'

'They're lucky to be alive.'

Bernie knocked back his brandy. 'Yeah, very lucky. I saw hundreds of planes circling over the docks. Terrible sight, it was, terrible. Anyway, I'd best be off. The missus sent me out for a few extras. I'll see if Harry is down the Prince's Head.'

'No need, here he is,' Winnie said, pointing to the door.

The sight of him made Winnie's heart pound. He breezed in looking as dapper as ever. The blue spots on his dickie bow tie matched the handkerchief in his jacket breast pocket. He was the only man in the pub who wore a suit. The others preferred a pullover and shirt.

'Harry, just the man,' Bernie said, sounding relieved.

'What can I do for you?' Harry asked. He ran a finger

over his dark pencil moustache and then doffed his trilby to Winnie.

'I'm going to need whatever you've got on offer.'

Harry's grey eyes lit up. 'Come with me, my man, let's have a chat in my office,' he said and led Bernie to his usual table in the corner.

Winnie sent Lucy over with a drink for Harry. The man conducted good business from that table and having Harry in the pub brought in more customers.

'After you've served Harry, pop out the back and make us a cuppa, there's a love.'

The door opened again and relief washed over Winnie. She'd never been so pleased to see Terence Card walk in. 'Thank Gawd,' she uttered, hoping that Terry would have news of Jan. 'Have you seen her? Have you seen my Jan? Is she all right?' Winnie asked, her words tumbling out.

'Yes, Win. She's fine. I borrowed the bakery van and popped over to the hospital. I only saw her for a minute. She was really busy and looked exhausted. She sends her love and said you're not to worry about her.'

'Oh, Terry, I can't tell you what that means to me,' Winnie said. A sob caught in her throat as she fought to hold back tears of joy. 'The poor girl, she must have seen some awful sights.'

Terry swallowed hard and lowered his eyes. 'It's not good over there, Win. The fires are still blazing. It chokes you, takes your breath away. One old dear was screaming about the rats.'

'The rats?'

'Yeah. The explosions and the fires apparently brought all the rats out. Strange, ain't it?'

'There's no words, love. Nothing can describe it. I thought

it was bad enough during the Great War and look how long that went on for. But this … the planes …' Winnie's words trailed off as she struggled to contain her emotions. If anyone had said that they weren't scared last night, they would have been lying. But Winnie had put on a brave face for Rachel and Lucy. Now, the news that Jan was unharmed had brought Winnie's feelings to the surface but she couldn't be seen crying behind the bar. 'Right, that'll do. I'll have no more talk of bombs and war in my pub today. Let 'em come. Let the Germans do their worst but they won't beat us and they won't break us.'

'Here, here, well said, Win,' Len chirped and raised his tankard. 'I'll drink to that.'

Hilda was next to come through the door and she walked across the pub to stand alongside Terry. 'Hello, you two. Glad to see you're both OK.'

'We're fine, love. Are you?'

'I ain't going to lie, I was in bits last night but I've pulled myself together now.'

'Did you go to the public shelter?'

'No. I hid under me bed.'

'People are saying that they expect the Germans will come back again. If they do, you really should get yourself to a proper shelter.'

'Yeah, I will, Win. I don't think I could stand another night alone under me bed like that.'

'Well, I'm glad you're all right, but I thought you would have been here earlier to see Rachel and Martha.'

'I would have been but I was busy with the WVS. Actually, I wanted to talk to you about that.'

'I'm all ears,' Winnie said, curious to know more.

'Well, with Jan off nursing now, I've found myself with plenty of time on my hands and you know that can be dangerous for me,' Hilda said, looking past Winnie and gesticulating towards the bottles of whisky.

Winnie knew the booze would always be a temptation for Hilda but she hoped the woman wouldn't let Rachel and the baby down. Hilda had given her word that she'd never drink again and had kept to it so far. 'You've done really well,' Winnie said.

'Yeah, I know. But I miss working with Jan. So, instead of sitting all day on my sewing machine making dresses, I've signed up with the Women's Reserve Volunteers. I had a few errands to run this morning and tomorrow I start on mending vests and trousers for our boys. There's even talk of me teaching the soldiers how to mend their own clothes,' Hilda said proudly.

'Good for you.'

'But do you think Rachel will mind? It means I won't be around so much during the day to help with Martha.'

'Don't worry, Hilda. Rachel is coping fine and now I've got Lucy to help behind the bar so Rachel doesn't need to be down here as much.'

'Lucy?'

'Yes, here she is,' Winnie said with a warm smile as the girl carried in two cups of tea from the back kitchen.

'Oh, hello,' Hilda greeted her. 'You look just like my Rachel.'

'This is Hilda,' Winnie told Lucy. 'She's Rachel's mum.'

'And Martha's gran,' Hilda added. 'Though you'll never hear Rachel call me "Mum". She thought I was her sister until about a year ago.'

Lucy looked taken aback at Hilda's revelation.

'And another thing. If I ever ask you for a whisky, don't serve me one and be sure to tell Winnie that I asked.'

Lucy looked confused so Winnie explained, 'Hilda doesn't drink ... anymore.'

'Well, nice to meet you, Lucy. I'd better go and break the news to my daughter,' Hilda said.

'She's joined the WVS,' Winnie informed Lucy as Hilda went to go upstairs.

'I'll probably have to do something for the war effort soon,' Lucy said.

'Let's just wait and see, eh, love.'

Bernie headed towards the door and called, 'See ya later' to Winnie. Harry was close behind him and threw Winnie a cheeky wink before he left. The gesture made Winnie blush. She felt ridiculous. After all, Harry was a cheeky chap and probably winked at everyone. But the man had a knack of making her feel special.

Minutes later, Harry returned, only now he had his son with him. Winnie wasn't pleased to see Errol. She had never liked him and never would. The young man had a nasty streak and was known to be violent. Errol was nothing like his father. He certainly didn't have Harry's charm or easy smile. And it was only last year that she'd had her own run-ins with Errol, who had been demanding money from her son. Mind you, after Winnie had discovered what David had done to Rachel and how he'd robbed the takings from the pub, she thought David probably deserved everything he got from Errol. The trouble was, it had been Winnie who had been left to clean up David's mess. Though she had to give credit where credit was due – Errol had been a model customer since Harry had been working from her pub.

Winnie served them as Lucy collected glasses. She saw Errol's eyes follow her new barmaid around the pub.

'Who's the new girl?' Errol asked his father.

'That's Lucy. But leave her be or Mrs Berry will have your guts for garters,' Harry answered.

Winnie placed their drinks on the bar and Harry winked at her again. She hoped her cheeks hadn't reddened as she sternly told Errol, 'That's right, I will. My barmaids are here to serve you drinks and that's it, nothing more.'

'All right, calm down. I was only asking,' Errol said.

'Oi, show some respect. That's no way to talk to Mrs Berry,' Harry told Errol.

Errol pulled his eyes away from Lucy to look at Winnie. With a sardonic smile and tone to his voice, he apologised.

Winnie busied herself washing the glasses that Lucy had collected. She could hear snippets of the conversation between Harry and Errol. They were discussing something about ration books and Errol didn't sound happy. There seemed to be some tension between them which she found unnerving. Errol towered over his father and Winnie thought that if the mood took him, he could easily knock Harry to the floor. It wasn't a fight that she would like to get between!

Errol's voice suddenly became louder, which caused Winnie to tense.

'I ain't a kid, Dad, so stop treating me like one,' he shouted.

Winnie looked over to see Errol slam his glass down on the bar and then storm off. She glanced at Harry. The man had his hands stretched on the bar and was shaking his head.

'Sorry about that. He's always been hot-headed.'

Winnie dried her hands and walked towards Harry. 'I know. Your lad has quite a reputation.'

'I've heard. He doesn't get it from me. He's got his mother's temper.'

'Hmm, I suppose it's that Spanish blood. Them foreigners from hot countries are quite fiery.'

'Yeah, something like that,' Harry said. He swigged several gulps of stout and then looked down at the floor.

Winnie got the impression that there was something that Harry wasn't saying and she had a good idea what it was. Years back, just before David had started school, a bloke had come into the Battersea Tavern looking for Carmen. Though he had said her name was Euphemia. It had stuck in Winnie's mind as it was such an unusual name. Anyway, he described Carmen to a tee. Someone told the fella where to find her. That evening, the same bloke returned to the pub. He'd burst through the door with a face like thunder and then drank several drinks. The alcohol loosened his tongue and he started shouting about Euphemia being a fraud and living a lie, denying her own family. He told anyone who would listen that her name wasn't Carmen. She wasn't Spanish but was the illegitimate child of a gypsy father. He said he was her brother and that he was disgusted at her for not showing up at their mother's funeral. No one had taken any notice of him and eventually Brian had thrown the bloke out. But Winnie had always known there was some truth in the man's ramblings. It made no difference to Winnie. She would never judge a woman for having a child out of wedlock. After all, she'd had one herself – her daughter, Alma, taken from her just minutes after she'd been born. And now her granddaughter, Martha, born to a mother without a husband. But Winnie thought

Carmen must be deeply ashamed of her past and where she'd come from. If the woman didn't have such a spiteful mouth, Winnie might have felt sorry for her. But she wondered what had made Carmen so bitter. She hadn't always been that way. Winnie could remember when Carmen had been kind and friendly. What had happened to change her so much? After all, it appeared that Carmen led a charmed life.

Her thoughts drifted back to Martha.

'You look deep in thought there,' Lucy said as she sidled up beside Winnie.

'I was just thinking about mothers and babies. I tell you what, after last night's shenanigans, I wouldn't be surprised if all those children who came back from the countryside get sent back there again.'

Lucy nodded emphatically. 'Yep, most likely. My three sisters were billeted to Norfolk but came back to my mum last month. I think you're right, Winnie. I reckon my mum will pack them off to Norfolk again.'

'It's a shame my Errol is too old to be evacuated,' Harry said with a chortle and he rolled his eyes.

'Was that Errol I saw leaving?' Lucy asked.

Winnie noticed a twinkle in the girl's eyes and hoped she wasn't sweet on him.

'Yeah, that's my son. He's a bit of a lady's man, so watch how you go with him,' Harry warned.

And there it was again. Winnie wasn't mistaken. Harry winked at her and she was sure that she saw something in his eyes. She couldn't quite describe what it was but there was definitely something there. Was he flirting?

Suddenly she found herself feeling flustered and she hurried off to serve Len another drink. She couldn't understand what had got into her lately. But there was something about Harry that made her stomach flip every time she saw him. She enjoyed his company and, if she was honest, she liked the attention from him too. But she knew she was being foolish and quickly chastised herself. *Stop being so stupid,* she thought, *Harry's a married man. And even if he weren't, he wouldn't be interested in you.* And apart from anything else, Winnie reminded herself that she was still married to Brian!

'I'll see you soon, Mum,' Lucy called over her shoulder as she walked up the short garden path from her mother's house.

Her mother stood on the tatty doorstep with her youngest daughter on her hip and waved Lucy off. 'You take care, dear. See you next week.'

Lucy was glad that the Battersea Tavern closed after Sunday lunch. It meant she could continue her normal routine of visiting her mother. Her mum had been shocked to hear that Lucy was working in a pub and horrified to discover that she was living with an unmarried woman and her baby. Lucy had tried to put her mother straight about the situation and had told her that Rachel was really nice. And Martha, well, she was the cutest little girl that Lucy had ever laid eyes on. Holding the baby had really pulled at her heartstrings and affirmed more than ever how much she yearned for a husband and child of her own. But no matter how much Lucy waxed lyrical about Rachel and Martha, Lucy's mother didn't want to hear it. Without even meeting Rachel, she'd decided that the girl must be loose. Lucy couldn't blame her mum for thinking that way. She had thought the same but now she felt awful for it and could see how small-minded she'd been. She knew that Winnie's son, David, was Martha's father but she didn't know where David was or why he wasn't around. She'd heard snippets of conversation and had gathered that David wasn't very well thought of. For now, Lucy didn't feel she knew Rachel well enough to ask any probing questions but she was sure she'd find out all about it in good time. It was just nice to have someone of her own age around, though she found Rachel to be quite boring. But Lucy didn't have any other friends. Carol, her so-called best mate, had talked about her behind her back and now hung about with Anne Caldwell. Well, good riddance to the pair of them.

The sun had almost set as Lucy turned the corner and approached the pub. It was an ominous building, the biggest in the street. Lucy had passed it many times but had never taken much notice. She'd never dreamed that she would be living in it! She thought Carol would be jealous. A pub was much more fun than the factory where she'd worked with Carol and Anne alongside Cheryl and Yvonne.

As Lucy felt in her coat pocket for the back-door key, she gasped in horror when the sound of the air-raid siren suddenly wailed into life. It shouldn't have been a surprise. Most of the customers in the pub that morning had said the Germans would bomb again. But Lucy hadn't expected them to return so soon!

She hurried in through the back door and called to Winnie and Rachel. They didn't answer so she guessed they must already be downstairs in the cellar. As she made her way there, she heard someone knocking heavily on the pub door. She stood for a moment and chewed her bottom lip, wondering if she should answer the door or call down to Winnie.

The knocking became more urgent, louder and faster. Lucy picked up the key from behind the bar and dashed through the pub. She unbolted the top and bottom locks before opening the door to find a young, good-looking man smiling at her.

'Hello, who are you?' he asked as his eyes roamed over her.

'I'm Lucy. I work here. Can I help you?'

'Yes, probably,' he answered and craned his neck to look over her shoulder. 'Excuse me,' he added and side-stepped her to get through the door.

'Erm – what do you think you're doing?' Lucy asked.

The man was in the pub now and walking towards the bar.

'You can't come in. We're closed. Please leave this instant.'

'It's all right. I've come to see my mum, Winnie. Where is she?'

'She'll be in the cellar. But you can't go down there,' Lucy answered in a panic. The sirens were still screaming. The Germans would be overhead at any minute. And now there was a strange man in the pub. He could be Winnie's son but what if he wasn't? 'You'll have to leave. Come back later,' she urged.

The man turned and looked at her. 'It's all right. My mum will be pleased to see me,' he said and headed towards the door that led down to the cellar.

Lucy rushed after him. 'Stop. I told you, you can't go down there. I'd like you to get out of Mrs Berry's pub immediately.' Her voice was firm and steady but Lucy could feel herself trembling. She wasn't sure if she was more scared of the Luftwaffe or of confronting this strange man. She went to pull on his arm but he had already opened the door and begun to descend the stairs.

Lucy closely followed him. 'I'm sorry,' she called ahead, 'I tried to stop him.'

The lighting in the cellar was quite dim but she saw a horrified expression on Winnie's face and the colour drained from Rachel's. Both women stared at the man in disbelief.

'Hello, Mum, Rachel,' he said, glancing from one to the other.

'David!' Winnie exclaimed. Her mouth hung open as she glared at him with wide eyes.

So, this was Martha's father, Lucy thought, as she realised that he hadn't been lying about his identity. But from the expression on Winnie's and Rachel's faces, it seemed that he wasn't a welcome sight.

'Have you missed me?' David asked in a mocking manner.

Winnie rose to her feet. 'Get out!' she spat. 'How dare you walk back in here like nothing happened. Go on, get out!'

'Whoa, hang on a minute, Mum. I'd like to meet my baby first. Boy? Girl?'

Lucy noticed that Rachel had pulled Martha closer to her chest and turned her away from David's prying gaze.

'You're having nothing to do with that child. I won't tell you again, you're not welcome here, David, so get out, or I'll send for the police.'

'You'd send your own son out onto the streets in the dark and during a bombing raid? Come on, Mum, it ain't safe outside.'

'Go to a public shelter. You ain't staying here. And as far as I'm concerned, you ain't no son of mine!'

'Ouch, that hurt,' David said and placed his hands over his heart. 'I thought you might have been a bit more pleased to see me. Look, I know I messed up, but I'm sorry. Give me another chance, eh? I've missed you, Mum.'

'More like you've missed my purse. That's it, ain't it? You've

49

run out of money so you thought you'd come back here with your tail between your legs to see what you could steal from me again. I ain't having it. Sling your hook and don't bother coming back.'

Winnie began to shove David towards the stairs. Lucy had to move out of the way.

'Get off, what do you think you're doing?' he moaned.

'Get out. Go on. Out,' Winnie said, pushing him away.

'All right, all right, get off me, I'm going. But just so you know, I'm not here for money. I've got a job, a good one, and my own place.' He was halfway up the stairs with Winnie in his wake.

'I don't want to hear it, David.'

'If a bomb lands on my head out there, you'll be sorry.'

'No, I won't.'

'It'll be on your conscience.'

'I can live with that,' Winnie answered coldly.

They were at the top of the stairs and then through the door. Lucy tried to listen but couldn't hear them. She looked at Rachel who appeared to have been holding her breath and now she let out a long sigh.

'Are you all right?'

Rachel swallowed hard. 'I can't believe he turned up like that.'

'Is that the first time you've seen him since Martha was born?'

'Yes. He ran off when he found out I was pregnant and he took the pub's takings with him.'

'Oh!'

'He's not a nice man. I hope he doesn't stay in Battersea.'

The cellar door opened and Winnie trudged back down the stairs. 'I got rid of him. What a bleedin' cheek!'

'I'm sorry, Winnie, I tried to stop him.'

'It's not your fault, love. He's gone for now but I doubt that'll be the last we see of him.'

Lucy was pleased that Winnie didn't blame her for allowing David in but she was shocked that Winnie had thrown him out while the air-raid sirens were wailing. He'd run off and left Rachel with an unborn child and had stolen from his mum but chucking him out like that, possibly to his death, well, it seemed a bit harsh. After all, David had apologised but Winnie hadn't accepted it. The woman seemed overly harsh with her son. Perhaps she wasn't quite as nice as Lucy had first thought and she wondered if Winnie had a swinging brick for a heart.

4

Winnie felt exhausted. She hadn't slept a wink and it wasn't
just the German bombers that had kept her awake. She'd
been pleased to see that, since David had left, no harm had
come to her son, but she couldn't believe that he'd had the
audacity to breeze back into their lives.

She looked across the kitchen table at Rachel. The girl
seemed unusually quiet and subdued, which didn't surprise
Winnie. She thought Rachel must still be in a state of
shock after unexpectedly coming face to face with David.
Throughout the night, Winnie had repeatedly told Rachel
that her son would never be welcome back in the Battersea
Tavern and had reaffirmed her vow again. 'My door will
always be open for anyone who needs a cup of tea, a blanket
or a hot meal. But I won't have David under my roof and
that's final,' she said firmly. 'Right, that said, let's get the doors
open downstairs. Rachel, give Lucy a hand to get the urn
up from the cellar. Then, Lucy, bring the blankets downstairs
from the airing cupboard. I shouldn't think we will need
them this morning but let's get prepared.'

With Martha sleeping soundly in her cot, the women

followed Winnie's instructions and Winnie trudged down the stairs and opened up the pub. It was 8.15 a.m., no alcohol would be served. But at least they could offer refuge and sympathy to anyone in need.

Winnie stepped outside and looked up and down the street. Everything appeared to be intact. She was grateful that the area around them had, so far, missed being damaged. But she'd heard on the wireless that incendiaries had caused fires in Tooting, Clapham, Brixton and Streatham. All night, for the second night running, bombs had rained down on London. Winnie thought about Jan. She doubted that Jan would have had any rest. Hundreds of people would have been taken to St Thomas's. There'd be burn victims, injuries from flying shrapnel and buildings collapsing. She didn't know how her daughter, as she always thought of her, had the stomach for it but she thought to herself, *Thank goodness for people like my Jan.*

Len came out from the corner shop and walked along the street towards her. He lived around the bend at the other end. Winnie noticed his limp was more pronounced than she'd seen before. She assumed his arthritis must be playing up.

'Good morning, Winnie. I went for me paper but they ain't got them in yet. I hope the printers ain't been bombed.'

'I don't know, but I heard that there's a lot of warehouses and factories near the docks that got hit.'

'Down that end of the street, you can see the smoke from the fires.'

'I'd rather not look, Len, it makes my blood run cold. Do me a favour. Put the word about that I'm open for anyone who needs a cuppa.'

'Will do, pet.'

Winnie sighed as Len plodded off. Everything seemed so normal around her yet it was only a few miles away that folk had lost their homes and their belongings. Many had lost their lives too. She'd always felt safe in Battersea and had never believed that the place would be worth bombing. She hadn't thought that there was much in the borough for the Germans to worry about. But her customers had said that the Jerries would come. Battersea Power Station would be a target and so would Clapham Junction railway station. There were some big factories and industries along York Road too – Garton's Glucose Factory, Morgan's Crucible Works, Price's Candles and the brewery and distillery. Not to mention the flour mills near the river Thames. The Germans weren't to know what went on in those big buildings and would likely try to blow them up. The thought terrified Winnie though she kept her fears to herself.

She pulled her cardigan around her body and folded her arms across her chest, keeping out the morning chill. She looked up and down the street again, wondering where David was. She guessed that he'd gone to stay with one of his friends, if he had any. But she knew she hadn't yet seen the last of him. It broke her heart to turn her back on her only son. But what else could she do? He'd shown himself to be just like his father. They said that the apple doesn't fall far from the tree and it was true with Brian and David. Winnie's foot tapped with frustration. She'd done everything for that boy. Perhaps that was the problem. Maybe she'd spoiled him. But she was adamant that she'd taught him right from wrong and what he'd done to Rachel had been very wrong indeed. No matter how much David begged, cried or screamed, Winnie knew that she had to remain firm. She loved her boy but she

54

couldn't forgive him. She was going to have a battle on her hands – David was a master of manipulation. But Winnie was determined to keep her heart hardened towards him. Even though, in truth, all she really wanted was to have him tucked up safely in his old bed upstairs.

Cheryl pushed in front of several women in the queue to join Yvonne, ready to clock on at the factory.

'Oi, get to the back,' Ada, shouted from behind.

'I ain't pushing in. Yvonne's been holding my place,' Cheryl called along the line.

The older woman was further back in the queue. Cheryl wasn't surprised that Ada had confronted her. The two had never got on. Ada was partial to gossiping and wasn't afraid to speak her mind. She often clashed with Cheryl, who had strong opinions of her own and would voice them freely.

Ada spoke again in a huffy tone. 'You're taking liberties, you are. Just cos you're a Hampton, it don't give you the right to do as you please.'

'Just ignore her,' Yvonne whispered.

Cheryl's lips pursed as she looked ahead and tried to contain her anger. Ada quite often made snide comments about her family. Cheryl put it down to jealousy. After all, while Ada and many like her were making do with meagre rations and utility clothing, Cheryl was enjoying the luxuries her father brought home. Even before the war, Cheryl had considered herself and her family to be a cut above the rest of the riff-raff of Battersea. They lived in a standard terraced house but it was decorated the nicest and they wore the smartest clothes, especially Errol in his smart suits. Her father saw to it that they were always well turned out.

Cheryl's ears pricked again at the sound of Ada's raised voice. The woman was talking loudly enough to ensure that everyone could hear her.

'Them Hamptons need bringing down a peg or two, if you ask me. The way they carry on, well, it ain't fair. Harry is flogging his black-market stuff and making a small fortune but it's no good to the likes of us. Good, hardworking folk like me and you can't afford the extortionate prices he charges. And what about Errol Hampton, eh? Why ain't he doing his bit? He looks fine, he should have enlisted, but he's swanning around like there ain't a war going on. He's a shirker, that's what he is, and I ain't too scared of him to say so.'

Cheryl felt Yvonne's hand on her arm but she couldn't hold back and quickly spun round to be faced with a sea of accusing eyes. All the women appeared to be looking at her for an answer. But Cheryl was reluctant to give them one. Why should she? What her family did was nothing to do with Ada or anyone else. Instead, she barked, 'Shut your mouth, Ada. You don't know what you're talking about.'

'Huh, I'm right. Your brother is a shirker and a coward. He should have enlisted when my Arthur did.'

'I said, shut your mouth! Or I'll come back there and shut it for you. It ain't none of your business, so poke your nosey beak out.'

'Typical! You all heard that. She threatened me. Well, like I said, I ain't scared of your brother and I certainly ain't worried about a little mouthy cow like you.'

Cheryl went to confront Ada but Yvonne grabbed her arm. 'Leave it, Cheryl. She just wants a reaction from you.'

'Yeah, and she's gonna bloody well get one,' Cheryl hissed and pulled her arm free from Yvonne's grip.

As she marched towards Ada, the line of women were quick to move out of her way. She stood in front of Ada, glaring angrily. Ada wasn't intimidated and eyed Cheryl from head to toe with a look of contempt. 'You Hamptons have always been the same. Your mother's got her nose so far stuck up her own backside, she must think the world stinks of her own muck. And you, well, you're just like her.'

Cheryl pulled her arm back in anticipation of swinging it round to give Ada a stinging slap across her cheek. But she was stopped abruptly by the sound of their supervisor's booming voice.

'Come on, you lot, what's the hold-up?' Mr Mullen called.

'Er, nothing, sir,' Carol answered from somewhere near the front of the queue.

'Good. Then hurry up and clock on and get to work.'

Cheryl leaned in towards Ada. 'You'll keep,' she whispered menacingly.

Ada smirked and replied, 'I'll be waiting.'

Cheryl made her way back to Yvonne. Her friend was shaking her head disapprovingly. 'You'll get sacked, if you're not careful,' she warned Cheryl.

'I don't care. I won't have anyone bad-mouth my family.'

'You shouldn't take any notice of Ada. She's always looking for a row; you know what she's like.'

Cheryl nodded to placate her friend but she had no intention of ignoring Ada and her big mouth. She thought it was about time that someone shut up the dreadful woman. And though Ada stood a good five inches over her and was twice as wide to boot, Cheryl was a Hampton and she wouldn't back down.

Just as she'd expected, the mood in the factory was very

subdued. There was none of the usual banter and laughter. Everyone seemed to be struggling to keep their eyes open. Two consecutive nights of air raids were already taking their toll. The morning dragged on with the monotonous work. It was a welcome relief when Mr Mullen sounded the bell for lunchtime.

'Shall we take a walk and eat our sandwiches in the yard?' Yvonne asked.

Cheryl could read her friend like a book. She knew that Yvonne's suggestion was a ruse to keep her out of the canteen and away from Ada. But she was so tired she readily agreed.

Outside, the young women sat on a bench. Cheryl was glad of the fresh air which woke her up a bit. Yvonne unwrapped her sandwich and wrinkled her nose at the questionable paste inside. 'What's in yours?' she asked.

'Egg. Would you like to share?'

'Yes please. This is only fit for the pigeons,' Yvonne answered. 'It's not my mum's fault. She tries hard to make the food last but my brother keeps helping himself to it. I've heard me mum having a go at him but you know what he's like. He takes no notice of her.'

Cheryl felt sorry for Yvonne. Her father had died seven years earlier leaving Yvonne's mum with four children to bring up. Yvonne was the oldest and the only girl. She'd been expected to help to look after her younger brothers and had done so without complaint. 'Tell you what, why don't you come round to my house after work. I'll get my mum to sort out a few bits for your mum.'

'Thanks, Cheryl, but we don't need charity.'

'It's not charity. Honestly, you should see what we've got at home. It's bursting at the rafters. I don't know what my dad has been up to, but he's even got stuff stashed under the floorboards in his bedroom. It's like Aladdin's cave. My mum will be glad to get rid of some things to give her a bit more space. We're almost falling over the stuff.'

'Are you sure?'

'Yes, of course I'm sure.'

'Thank you. Will Errol be home?'

'I doubt it,' she answered and hid a smile. Yvonne was obviously still carrying a torch for her older brother.

'What Ada said this morning, you know, about Errol not enlisting. I know it's nothing to do with me but I have wondered.'

'He's medically unfit but don't ever mention it. He doesn't like people knowing his business.'

'What's wrong with him?'Yvonne asked, sounding alarmed. But then she added quickly, 'Sorry, I shouldn't pry.'

'He's got a hernia and wears a truss. But for Gawd's sake don't tell anyone.'

'I won't, I swear.'

Cheryl was glad her brother wasn't fighting with the British army. Next to Yvonne, he was the only other friend she had and she couldn't stand the thought of anything awful happening to him. She finished her half of the egg sandwich and then told Yvonne, 'We'd better get back.'

Cheryl sat at her bench and got on with her work.Yvonne sat beside her and Carol opposite, next to Anne. They were all about the same age and got on well together. Carol and Anne were best friends just like Cheryl and Yvonne. Normally, on a Monday, they'd be swapping tales of what they'd been up to at the weekend but today was different. The attack on the inhabitants of London seemed to be the only thing on anyone's mind. Cheryl was pleased that the friends on her bench didn't want to talk about it and preferred to sit in silence.

An hour or so had passed when Cheryl felt something unexpectedly hit the back of her head. She looked down at the floor and saw a piece of rubber. She didn't take any notice and carried on working. But then something landed on her head again and she saw another piece of rubber bounce off her and land on the floor nearby. This time, Cheryl glanced over her shoulder and instantly knew that Ada was trying her upmost to antagonise her. The woman was staring back at Cheryl with a wicked sneer on her face. Cheryl looked across to Mr Mullen but he was engrossed in his paperwork. And then Ada blatantly lobbed another piece of rubber at Cheryl, which hit her on the forehead.

'Ignore her, she ain't worth it,' Yvonne advised.

Cheryl was about to leap out of her seat but Yvonne was right. Ada wasn't worth losing her job over. If she rushed over to Ada's bench now, it would be Cheryl, not Ada, who would be in trouble with Mr Mullen. She gritted her teeth and turned back to her work.

'I can't stand Ada and her cronies. They're mean,' Carol whispered.

Anne leaned forward and said quietly, 'She used to pick on me when I first started working here. But, one day, I was outside Woolworths and I bumped into Ada. She started having a go at me, saying I didn't dress appropriately. My mum came out of the shop and gave her a right mouthful. Ada ain't said a word to me since.'

'She's a bully,' Carol added.

'I'll get her. I swear I will,' Cheryl mumbled under her

breath. And she meant it. Bully or not, Cheryl would bide her time and would glean great pleasure in wiping that smug smile off Ada's face once and for all.

As soon as Harry heard the shocking news, his heart sank. Poor Winnie, he thought. He knew that she would be devastated when she found out, though he doubted that she'd been made aware of it yet. He was riding his motorbike at top speed to get to the Battersea Tavern as fast as he could. When he pulled up outside, he was surprised to find it open at this early time of the morning.

Harry climbed off his bike and took a deep breath before walking in. He wasn't looking forward to breaking this news to Winnie and hoped she wouldn't crumple. He wasn't very good at dealing with upset women.

The pub smelt musty, of old tobacco and stale beer. Funny, he'd never really noticed it before. Winnie was standing behind the bar. Lucy was at the end of the bar pouring cups of tea from an urn.

'Morning, Harry,' Winnie chirped with a beaming smile.

Harry gulped. The woman always had a cheery greeting for her customers, regardless of the circumstances. But what he was about to impart would change all that and Winnie's smile would likely change to tears. 'Morning,' he replied and then told her firmly. 'Don't panic, but I need you to get your hat and coat and come with me.'

'Why?'

'Go and get your hat and coat and I'll explain on the way.'

'On the way to where? You needn't think I'm getting in that sidecar thing again.'

'Please, Winnie.'

'I ain't budging until you tell me what this is about.'

Harry knew the woman could be stubborn. He looked over to Lucy. 'Can you get Mrs Berry's hat and coat please, sweetheart.'

Winnie was looking confused. 'I want to know what's going on?' she demanded, her hands now on her wide hips.

Harry knew he had no choice but to tell her straight. 'I'm taking you over to Westminster. St Thomas's Hospital took a hit last night. But try not to worry. We'll go there right now and check on your Jan. I'm sure she's fine.'

Winnie's red cheeks paled and, for a moment, Harry thought that she might faint. Lucy appeared with her coat and hat.

'Put your coat on. Let's go,' Harry instructed calmly. He turned to Lucy, 'Keep things running here. Rachel can help if you need her.'

Lucy nodded and helped Winnie on with her coat.

'A bomb ... on the hospital ...' she mumbled, as if what Harry had just told her was only just sinking in.

'Yes. But it'll be all right,' he said, hoping to reassure her. But in truth, he couldn't promise that it would be and he feared the worst.

Outside, Harry helped Winnie climb into the sidecar. She was quite a large lady and only just fitted in. Her lips were tight as she stared directly ahead. Harry couldn't imagine what must be going through her mind. He knew how he'd feel if it was his daughter who'd been caught up in an explosion. Cheryl was a feisty little thing with her mother's temper but would always be his precious little girl. He couldn't stand the thought of anything like this happening to her. For Winnie's sake, he hoped more than anything that Jan had been spared from any harm.

They sped through Battersea and towards Westminster. As they approached the Thames, they could clearly see the smoke from the fires on the other side of the river. From their viewpoint, it looked as though the whole of East London was alight! Harry's heart hammered. It wasn't boding well for Jan.

It took them a while to navigate through the bomb-damaged streets. They had to drive slowly to avoid the rubble from collapsed buildings which was strewn across the roads. The emergency services were everywhere and working with an army of volunteers. Some people were wandering around aimlessly and looking dazed and shocked. Others were dashing from here to there, offering help where they could. As Harry approached Westminster Bridge, he could see that the nurses' home had taken a direct hit. The front of the building was gone, exposing tall walls on either side and showing evidence of where floors had once been. Most of the bricks and cement now lay on the ground and covered one side of the bridge. Harry glanced at Winnie. Silent tears were streaming down her face. He doubted that she was crying because of the wind in her eyes.

A policeman stepped in front of the motorbike and waved them down. Harry came to a stop and the policeman told them that they couldn't drive any further. Harry helped Winnie from the sidecar. He could feel her body trembling. They both stood and stared at what was left of the nurses' home. Men and women, some black with soot from head to toe, were slowly moving bricks, passing them along from one to the other. Harry could taste the acrid dust that hung in the air.

'Oh, my Gawd, my Jan could be buried under that lot!'

'Try not to worry, Winnie. She might be perfectly safe and working inside the hospital. Come on, let's see what we can find out.' He placed his hand on the back of Winnie's arm and gently urged her towards the fallen building.

A man beckoned to them and asked, 'Can I help you?' He had a tin helmet on and an arm band indicating that he was an air-raid warden.

'We're looking for someone. Jan Board. She's a nurse and this is her mother,' Harry answered.

'Oh, er, right. Best you go into the hospital and check. They've got a list.'

'A list? What sort of list?' Winnie asked.

The warden's eyes were downcast when he answered, 'Of the dead and injured.'

Winnie's hand flew to her mouth and she gasped.

'It's all right,' Harry soothed. 'There's no reason to think that Jan's name will be on it.'

'There's every reason! Look at that building. My Jan could have been in there!'

'But she might not have been. Tell you what. You wait here, I'll go and see about this list.'

'No. I'm coming with you,' Winnie said and she sniffed.

As they strode purposely ahead, Harry thought how surreal this seemed. If it weren't for the impressive sight of Big Ben and the Houses of Westminster in the background, the area would have been almost unrecognisable. He shuddered to think how many people might still be buried alive and prayed that they'd find survivors under the mess of twisted metal, bricks and shattered glass.

A nurse in a surprisingly white, crisp apron stood near

some temporary bollards that had been placed near the edge of the debris from the collapsed part of the building. She had a clipboard in her hand and was in conversation with a fire warden. Winnie rushed towards them and Harry followed.

'I'm looking for my daughter,' Winnie blurted. 'Jan Board. She's a nurse. Have you seen her?'

The nurse and the policeman exchanged an ominous look.

'Well? Do you know where my daughter is?' Winnie pressed.

The nurse placed her hand on Winnie's arm and offered a look of sympathy. Harry immediately knew that she was about to divulge bad news.

'I'm sorry to tell you this, but we think that Jan may be trapped in the building. They're doing everything they can to free her.'

'Trapped – in there?' Winnie asked, turning to point at the wreckage.

The nurse nodded. Suddenly, Winnie's legs seemed to buckle. Harry and the fire warden were quick to respond and managed to support her before she fell to the ground.

'Take her inside and get her a cup of tea,' the nurse told the fire warden.

'Come with me, dear,' he gently urged.

'No. No. I'm staying here. I need to be here for Jan, you know, when they dig her out. Harry – Harry, go and help them. Go and help them get my Jan out.'

'Yes, Winnie, of course I will. But let's sit you down some-where first, eh?'

'I'm fine,' she answered stoutly. 'Just do what you can to help them.'

Harry was impressed at how she'd pulled herself together.

He wasn't sure that he would be so strong if it were Cheryl buried in the debris. He went off to join the line of weary-looking men and women who were meticulously moving a ruined building, literally brick by brick. He glanced over at Winnie. The woman was standing with her shoulders back and her chin jutting forward, a look of determination on her face. It was clear that she wouldn't accept that Jan could be dead and Harry hoped beyond all hope that they would pull her out alive.

5

Lucy felt that she hadn't had a moment to herself but she didn't mind. She'd worked single-handedly all morning and found the time had flown by. Each customer had asked about Winnie's whereabouts and had seemed genuinely concerned on hearing about Jan. Lucy had thought it was quite touching, but she wondered if Winnie's loyal customers had any idea about how hard the woman could be. She'd witnessed how Winnie had thrown her own son out onto the street during an air raid. Lucy had thought the act to be quite heartless. After all, how bad could David be? Rachel must once have been enamoured with him, enough to have gone to bed with him. She thought Rachel was stupid to have slept with him out of wedlock but had to admit that David was very dishy! There was something about him that left her curious. She wanted to know more and couldn't believe he was as bad as Winnie and Rachel had portrayed him.

Lucy checked the clock. It was almost closing time and there'd still been no word from Winnie. Most of the customers had drifted out, only Len remained seated at the end of the bar in his usual place.

She was busy wiping out some ashtrays when she heard a 'Psst' from behind her.

Lucy turned to see Rachel peeping her head through the door that lead to the passageway and upstairs flat.

'Have you seen David?' Rachel asked in a whisper.

'No, he's not been in.'

Rachel sighed with relief. 'Thank goodness. But I'm certain he'll be back.'

Lucy shrugged. She didn't really understand why Rachel was so worried about seeing him. In fact, she hoped to bump into him but not in the pub under the watchful eyes of Rachel and Winnie.

'I'm getting really worried about Jan. I thought Winnie would have been back by now.'

'Terry came in earlier. He'd heard about the hospital and was heading straight there. At least Winnie won't be alone. She'll have Harry and Terry with her. How are you? I know Jan was your friend.'

'*Is* my friend. Please don't refer to her as if she's dead,' Rachel snapped.

'Sorry ... I didn't mean for it to come out like that.'

'No, it's all right. I'm sorry. I'm just worried sick about her and I shouldn't have spoken to you like that.'

'It's understandable. I'm closing up now. Shall we have a cup of tea upstairs?'

'Yes, I'll put the kettle on.'

Lucy offered a kind smile to Rachel and hoped that Rachel wouldn't see that it lacked sincerity. She didn't really want to be a shoulder for Rachel to cry on. She would have much preferred to go for a walk and possibly run into David. Still, there was no rush as Rachel and Winnie seemed to think that

David wasn't going away any time soon. She was sure that their paths would cross again and she was looking forward to it. Mind you, she'd be quite happy to see that Errol again too. He'd been just as attractive as David but she didn't like the idea of him being a lady's man. She knew his sort and had heard of his reputation. Though, looking at the way he dressed, Errol could be quite a catch!

Harry tucked into the liver and bacon Carmen had cooked, savouring every mouthful of the rich flavour. He would have enjoyed it all the more if he wasn't eating with his wife's scrutinising glare on him.

'I still don't see why you had to stay there all morning. And the state of your shoes and coat! They're ruined. Don't get me wrong, I feel sorry for Winnie, but, let's face it, Jan isn't really her daughter,' Carmen said coldly.

'Not by blood, but she loves the girl as if she were. What was I supposed to do? Just drive off and leave her there all alone?'

'Winnie isn't your responsibility. I'm sure there were plenty of people around; she'd hardly have been alone and Terry was there.'

'Christ, Carmen, you can be bloody heartless sometimes!'

'And you can be too flamin' soft, especially with our Cheryl. She had my sewing machine out yesterday and took all her skirts up a good two inches. She's asking for trouble.'

'Leave it out, woman, it's just the fashion. She'll be wearing trousers next, you watch.'

'Over my dead body! I won't have any daughter of mine wearing trousers. It's not ladylike,' Carmen said and tutted.

'Come off it, love. The women are working on the buses and trams, in the factories and all sorts. Things have changed.'

'The sooner this war is over, the better. Then things can go back to how they were.'

'I wouldn't count on that happening. From what I've seen, the young ladies like their new roles. Any chance of another cuppa?'

Carmen snatched Harry's cup from his hand and poured more tea from the pot. 'I'd appreciate a bit more support from you where Cheryl is concerned. Trust me, Harry, the girl needs keeping in line for her own good.'

Harry understood why his wife was so strict with Cheryl – Carmen didn't want her family history to repeat itself. She'd lived her life with the stigma of knowing her mother wasn't married to her gypsy father and she didn't want the same fate for Cheryl's children. But Carmen rarely showed her softer side to Cheryl and never offered any explanation for her harshness. Perhaps it would be better if Cheryl knew the truth and would then understand that her mother had her best interests at heart. But Carmen would do her nut if the reality about her past was ever mentioned. His wife would rather come over as an overbearing and stern mother than allow her children to know the circumstances of her birth.

'Are you listening to me, Harry?'

Carmen's voice broke into his thoughts and he answered, 'Yes, sweetheart. I'll keep an eye on Cheryl. And I'll have a word with Errol too, tell him to make sure that there's no unwanted attention around his sister.'

'I've already told him he's to keep any blokes in uniform away from Cheryl. I've seen plenty of young men full of bravado and looking dashing in their khakis. A girl's eye could easily be turned.'

'Turn your eye, did they?' Harry asked jokingly.

'Don't be ridiculous. An old woman like me wouldn't be looking at young men.'

'You're not old and you can still turn heads,' Harry said with a cheeky grin, winking at his wife.

'Don't be daft. That boat sailed a long time ago.'

'Oi, don't talk about my wife like that. She was a stunner when I met her and she still is.' Harry was pleased to see that his comments softened Carmen's face and her cheeks flushed a little. She even smiled which was rare these days.

'You're so full of it, Harry,' Carmen said, her tone warm.

When she reached across the table for his empty plate, Harry placed his large hand over her dainty one. His eyes locked with hers and he said sincerely, 'I don't tell you often enough, but I love you, girl. You know that, don't you?'

Carmen pulled her hand away and looked flustered. She jumped from her seat and went to the sink. Keeping her rod-straight back to Harry, she answered, 'Yes. I know.'

Today's events with Jan had made Harry realise how fragile life could be and how quickly it could be snuffed out. He'd said his piece. If anything untoward should happen to him, Carmen would at least know that she was loved. Though he had hoped for a bit more of an enthusiastic response. Granted, he hadn't expected Carmen to throw her arms around his neck and smother him in kisses. She'd never been a demonstrative woman and all passion in the bedroom had stopped years ago. Carmen had rebuked all his efforts, leaving him feeling frustrated and rejected. He supposed that he couldn't blame his wife for turning her back to him every night; he probably deserved it after what he'd done, but he'd hoped she would have forgiven him by now. And if Harry was honest, he wasn't sure that his wife had ever enjoyed a bit of 'how's your father'. It had always felt as if she'd been performing a duty. But they had gained Cheryl from it and his daughter had brightened his world. And he'd always have his other outlets for his needs. His mind drifted back again to Winnie and Jan. He hoped Winnie had had some good news by now. The thought of the woman's heart breaking left Harry feeling sick to his stomach.

'Oh, Terry, look at the state of your hands!' Winnie exclaimed as she peered from one of his hands to the other. His fingertips were grazed and swollen and blood oozed from numerous small cuts. He'd spent hours shifting bricks in the search for Jan, yet they still hadn't uncovered her.

Terry glanced down. 'Soft baker's hands, these. But once we've rescued Jan, I'm signing up, Win.'

'No, Terry, why on earth would you do that?' she asked, mortified at the thought.

'Look at what the Jerries are doing to us. I can't stand by any longer and watch. I've got to do my bit.'

'But you do, Terry. You volunteer for warden duties three nights a week.'

'It's not enough, Win. My mind is made up but I'll marry Jan before I go. Anyway, I just stopped for a minute to make sure you're all right?'

'Yes, love, I'm coping. There's a Women's Institute van over the road. Shall I get you a cuppa?'

'No, thanks. I'll get back to the search. You're sure you're OK?'

'Yes. You get on, find our Jan,' Winnie answered, her voice breaking as a sob caught in her throat.

The sun had moved across the sky and would be setting soon, yet there'd still been no sign of Jan, despite the heroic efforts of twenty or so men and women. Someone had brought a chair out from the hospital for Winnie to sit on. Cups of tea had been brought to her throughout the day and she'd even been offered a sandwich. Winnie had politely declined. She couldn't entertain the thought of food. Instead, a tight knot turned and twisted in her stomach. Surely they would find Jan soon.

Winnie tried to push the images from her mind but she kept finding herself imagining Jan under the rubble, terrified in the dark, all alone and struggling with the pain of the weight of the debris on top of her. But at least that awful thought was better than the alternative. Stop it, she told herself. She wouldn't allow herself to think that Jan could be dead. The thought was too harrowing. Though as the hours drifted by, the hope of pulling her out alive was slowly fading.

Suddenly, there was a flurry of activity and everyone rushed to one place. Winnie jumped to her feet and craned her neck. She wanted to walk over, to get closer, but her legs wouldn't move.

A man shouted to a nearby policeman. 'We've found someone!'

Winnie's pulse raced. It had to be Jan, it just had to be! 'Please, God, let her be alive,' she whispered as her pent-up emotion surfaced and her eyes welled with unshed tears.

The policeman hurried across to help the men, who were working frantically now. Hope of finding a survivor had spurred them on. Winnie's shaking legs finally worked and she approached, desperate to see her daughter but fearful of what she might find. With her eyes fixed on the scene in front of her, she stumbled on a brick, cursing as her ankle went over but unaware of the pain. She managed to stay on her feet and walked on, clutching her handbag so tightly to her chest that her knuckles went white.

Through the crowd, Winnie caught a glimpse of Terry and cried out in panic when she saw him drop to his knees. 'Oh, God, no, no, no, please, no!' she screamed and then picked up her pace, almost running now, tripping again as she clambered over the debris, grazing her knee on a chunk of concrete. Breathless, she reached the group of workers and pushed her way through but stood back from where Terry was on his knees.

Winnie couldn't make sense of what she was seeing. Terry had a hold of something that was poking through the bricks and dust. Was it a hand? Jan's hand? She didn't want to ask the question, terrified of what the answer might be, but she had to know and managed to stammer, 'My girl … Jan – is – is – is she dead?'

Terry looked up at her, his blue eyes wet with tears. 'She's alive, Win. Jan is alive!'

6

The following day, Winnie returned to the hospital to be with Jan, leaving Lucy to run the pub. She'd managed to get through another shift without any help from Rachel, who was still hiding away from David. So far, he hadn't returned again to the Battersea Tavern and none of Winnie's customers had seen him in the area. Lucy was beginning to think that she might never run into him again and couldn't help feeling disappointed.

She was hoping that once Len left, she could close, albeit twenty minutes early. But her hopes were dashed when two middle-aged men walked in and came to the bar. One smacked his lips together and asked for two halves of mild whilst the other said hello to Len and enquired after his health.

'There you go, gentlemen,' Lucy said as she placed their drinks on the counter.

'Thanks. Where's Winnie?'

'She's visiting her daughter in hospital,' Lucy answered.

'Jan? Nothing serious, I hope?'

'She was caught up in a bomb blast. She had to be dug

out of a fallen building, but luckily she wasn't seriously hurt, or worse.'

'Blimey, the poor love. Is that why David is back in Battersea?'

'You've seen him?' Lucy asked with more urgency in her voice than she'd have liked.

'Yeah, just a half-hour ago. He was heading towards Clapham Junction.'

'Did he say anything?'

'No, we didn't stop for a chat. Between you and me, I can't stand the bloke but I'd never let Winnie hear me say that. He's not back here to see Jan, then?'

'No, definitely not. Do you know where he might be staying?'

'Haven't got a clue and couldn't care less. But if I see him again, I'll find out what I can. You'll be wanting to close shop so we'll get on our way. Give my best to Winnie. I'm Bill, by the way, from the market. Me and the wife have got a dress stall.'

'Ah, yes, I thought I recognised you from somewhere. I'll tell Winnie that you called in. See ya.'

Bill and his mate departed and Len left shortly afterwards. Lucy couldn't wait to lock the door behind them. She sneaked up the stairs and grabbed her coat, hoping to avoid Rachel. She liked the girl well enough but found her a bit of a bore and didn't want to be lumbered with keeping her company for the rest of the afternoon. No, she had better things to do, Lucy thought with a wry smile, and quietly closed the back door behind her.

Clapham Junction bustled with shoppers. She hadn't expected to see it so busy, especially after the nightly attacks, but it seemed that Londoners were made of stern stuff. Throngs of people passed her, but, so far, there'd been no sign of David. She tried to imagine where he could be but couldn't think what business he might have in and around the shops. After over an hour of mooching around, Lucy was beginning to think that she was wasting her time and began to head back towards the Battersea Tavern. Suddenly, she was sure that she saw David step out of a tobacconist's. She was about to call out his name but that might seem a little too keen. Instead, she picked up her pace to try and catch up with him.

David stopped on the kerb, ready to cross the street. This was Lucy's opportunity. Her heart hammered; she was almost beside him.

'Oh, hello again,' she said nonchalantly with a flick of her hair.

David seemed to take a moment to recognise her, and then replied with a curt, 'Wotcha.'

'I'm Lucy, I work in the pub.'

'I know who you are,' he answered.

He showed no sign of being in the least bit pleased to see her and started to cross the street. Lucy walked briskly alongside him. 'Are you staying nearby?' she asked casually, fishing for something to say.

'Yes, not far. Why? Are you spying for my mum?'

'No, of course not. Look, I can see that there's some sort of problem between you and your mum but it's nothing to do with me and none of my business. I just work in the pub and get a room thrown in cheap. That's all.'

'You've not heard about me, then? They haven't blackened

77

my name and told you about Rachel? And about me robbing the pub?'

'They may have mentioned some things but, like I said, it's nothing to do with me. To be honest, I thought your mum was mean, throwing you out like she did; it wasn't safe. I'm pleased to see that no harm came to you.'

David looked round at her now and raised his eyebrows. 'Was you worried about me?' he asked with a dazzling smile.

'I was, actually.'

His blue eyes held her gaze until Lucy pulled away from his long stare.

'There's a café up the road. Would you like a drink? You can tell me all about how you came to be working for my mum.'

'Yeah, all right, I'll have a drink with you, but I'm sure we can find something better than your mum to talk about,' Lucy answered.

She gave David a teasing smile. She didn't care that he'd stolen from his mother and reasoned that he must have had good cause to. She wasn't bothered that he was the father of Rachel's baby. Rachel was foolish to have given herself to him without a ring on her finger. It seemed to her that David had been misunderstood by his mother and Rachel. From what Lucy had heard, they'd ganged up against him, and Hilda had too. He didn't stand a chance against the witches! But Lucy was willing to give him the chance that she believed he deserved. Butterflies fluttered in her stomach and when his hand accidently brushed against hers, she felt a jolt pass through her, leaving her tingling and wanting more. Lucy Berry, she thought wistfully. She liked the sound of that!

★

Cheryl left the factory with her arm linked through Yvonne's. 'Cor, I'm glad today is over with. It's only Tuesday and I'm worn out. If the Germans come back again tonight, I don't think I'll last until the end of the week.'

Yvonne nodded in agreement. 'You can say that again. My little brothers have been a nightmare. Mum won't go to the public shelter again because Edmund screamed the place down. We couldn't shut him up, it was awful. So last night, Mum got under the tin bath with him and me and Joey slept in the cupboard under the stairs. I know Joey was trying to be brave but he kept waking up after having bad dreams.'

'Kids don't understand. Edmund's only eight, bless him; you can't blame him for being scared of being dragged into the shelter with everyone. What about Ray, was he all right?'

'Ray's thirteen now and thinks he's a man. He's on about running away and signing up, the silly sod. He sat on guard last night watching for incendiaries, in case the house caught fire. He's a good kid.'

'They're all good kids. Your mum won't change her mind about having them billeted?'

'No, she won't hear of it. You know what she's like. Since me dad died, she likes to keep us all close. And by the way, thanks for the bags of food. She was over the moon and said it was like Christmas had come early.'

'You're welcome. There's plenty more where that came from. I know my mum can be a right cow sometimes but she's ever so generous.'

'She's a very kind lady.'

Cheryl had never heard anyone call her mother *kind*. It wasn't a word she'd have associated with her mum but Carmen had always been nice to Yvonne and Yvonne's family.

Maybe her mum felt sorry for them, but her empathy never extended to the rest of the poor families living in poverty around them. In fact, Cheryl would go so far as to say that, with the exception of Yvonne, nobody else liked her mum. 'Well, I don't know about you, but I've had enough of all this doom and gloom. We should cheer ourselves up. How about we go to the dance on Saturday? Me, you, Carol and Anne.'

'Are you sure it's still on? I think it may have been cancelled cos of the bombing.'

'It's been moved to the afternoon. So, how about it?'

'I'd love to but I'm not sure.'

'Oh, go on, Yvonne. It'll be a laugh. We could all do with that!'

'All right, I suppose so, but I'll have to be careful about how much I spend.'

'Don't worry about that. We'll find ourselves some nice young men to treat us.'

'Will Errol go to the dance?' Yvonne asked.

'I doubt it. It's not really his cup of tea. But I'll mention it. You can borrow my blue dress, if you like? And I'll get you some stockings from my dad. You won't need to be using any gravy browning on your legs.'

'Thanks, Cheryl, that's really nice of you. I love your blue dress, but are you sure you won't want to wear it?'

'I'm sure. I've got myself a knockout red one. Anyway, that's what friends are for.' Cheryl secretly hoped that if Yvonne wore her figure-flattering blue dress, she might attract the attention of a man. Someone who would distract Yvonne from wasting her thoughts and hopes on Errol. As nice as her friend was, with her mousy-brown straight hair and brown eyes that were too wide apart, she wasn't the prettiest of young women. And to make matters worse, Yvonne had a nervous habit of chewing her nails, which were right down to the wick. Cheryl knew that her brother would never be interested in Yvonne. She thought it was a shame really. She'd have liked Yvonne for a sister-in-law but there was no chance of that ever happening. And to add insult to injury, Cheryl had an inkling that Stephanie Reynolds was back on the scene and that Errol was seeing her again. She couldn't stand the woman.

'I'm feeling quite excited about it now,' Yvonne said.

'We could all meet in the Battersea Tavern,' Cheryl suggested, smiling.

'I'd rather come to your house and we can go to the pub together. I wouldn't have the nerve to walk in the pub by myself.'

'Great, we can do each other's hair,' Cheryl said enthusiastically. Her mind was already working on what she'd do to Yvonne's hair to glam her up. Her best friend would be the belle of the ball by the time Cheryl had finished with her. *Watch out, lads,* she thought, *here comes Yvonne!*

'I can't believe you're sitting up and talking,' Winnie gushed as she sat beside Jan's hospital bed.

'I'm very lucky.'

'Cor, not 'alf! But I still think you should come home for a few weeks and recuperate properly. I don't think you need to be rushing back to work.'

Jan sighed. 'I wish that were true but you've seen it here. They're struggling to keep up with the amount of injured people being rushed through the doors. I'm needed back at work as soon as possible. All hands on deck.'

Winnie couldn't argue with Jan. It was true. The hospital was stretched to its limits with bomb-blasted victims. But Winnie worried that Jan was pushing herself too hard. 'Won't you reconsider, even for just a couple of days?'

'I can't. I'd feel awful sitting with my feet up and knowing that I could be helping to save lives here.'

Now it was Winnie who sighed. 'Take no notice of me, love. I'm just being selfish. You're doing wonderful work here and this is where you should be. Changing the subject, has – erm – Terry said anything?'

'About what?'

'Oh, I don't know, nothing specific,' Winnie answered. She tried to hold back from beaming with delight but couldn't.

Her big smile must have given her thoughts away and as if reading her mind, Jan cautiously asked, 'Is Terry going to ask me to marry him?'

'I couldn't possibly say.'

'Oh my goodness, he is, isn't he! Tell me, Mum, I know you know. Is Terry going to propose to me?'

'Well, if he does, it's not before time!'

'Oh, oh my. Oh.'

'Don't you go letting on that I let the cat out of the bag.'

'I won't, I shall be the soul of discretion. I can't believe it! What did he say? When is he going to ask me?'

Winnie chuckled. She found it delightful to see Jan smiling after the terrible experience she'd been through. Jan hadn't said, but Winnie knew her daughter must have been scared for her life, buried under all the rubble. And even through her cuts and bruises, Jan's smile lit up Winnie's world. 'I'm not sure when he's going to ask you, love, but I think nearly losing you scared him half to death. I take it you're going to say yes?'

'Of course I am! Oh, Mum, I'm so happy, I could cry! My life has changed so much in the past year. I would never have dreamed it could be this good. If it wasn't for the war ... well ...'

'I know. But war or no war, we'll have a smashing wedding and a proper celebration in the pub.'

A very uppity-looking nurse walked along the ward and reminded people that visiting time was almost over.

'I'd best be off, love, but I'll be back tomorrow. Terry will be popping in this evening to see you. Remember, you mustn't say a word.'

'I won't, promise. But I hope he doesn't ask me when I'm in here. Look at the mess I'm in!'

'You're still beautiful and Terry obviously thinks so too. Now, get some rest. I'll see you tomorrow.'

After giving Jan a gentle kiss on her cheek, Winnie trudged along the ward, trying to avert her eyes from the injured patients in their beds. She supposed these people were the lucky ones. At least they were alive. Hundreds weren't and now Winnie feared that Hitler was going to continue his attack on London. She shuddered and pushed the thought away. Then as she came out of the hospital, she was surprised to see a familiar face sitting astride his motorbike and waving in her direction. Immediately, her pulse quickened.

'Harry, what are you doing here?' she asked as she buttoned her coat against the cool breeze.

'I came to give you a lift home.'

'That was very thoughtful of you, but don't you have better things to be doing?'

'No, not really. It's no trouble for me. Saves you traipsing across London on the trolleybus. Climb on board.'

Winnie eyed the sidecar with caution. She'd ridden in it a couple of times now and hadn't found the experience either comfortable or enjoyable. But she supposed it was convenient and she was grateful to Harry for going out of his way.

Harry got off his bike and came round to help Winnie manoeuvre herself. When he held her hand, the feelings it provoked left her too embarrassed to even glance at him. Once seated, she mumbled, 'Thank you.'

Thankfully, Harry didn't seem to notice that she was behaving strangely and he sped off towards Battersea. Throughout the journey, Winnie wrestled with her thoughts. She felt so silly for getting herself in a tizz about Harry, especially at her age. Though she wasn't an old woman yet and still had plenty of years left in her. There was no doubt that the man had awakened passions in her that she hadn't felt in ages. Once again, Winnie reminded herself that she was still married to Brian and Harry was married to Carmen.

When they arrived at the Battersea Tavern, Harry helped Winnie out of the carriage.

'Thanks ever so much for the lift,' she said, still flustered and avoiding eye contact. She stood on the pavement and straightened her coat. 'I think I'm getting used to that thing,' she added with a chuckle.

'You're always welcome, Winnie, you only have to ask. I can pick you up in the morning, if you like, and run you back to the hospital?'

'No, it's fine, thanks. I'll get the bus. You've been very generous but I'm sure you've got better things to do than running me around.'

'It's no bother.'

'No, really,' Winnie answered. She was grateful for Harry turning up at the hospital but she didn't want to take advantage of his kind ways.

'Right you are, but I'll come and pick you up again after visiting hours, no arguments.'

Before Winnie could protest, Harry had climbed back on his bike and was waving goodbye. She watched him ride off with a sinking feeling in her heart. Of all the men for her to fall for, how could she have been so stupid as to have allowed it to be Have-it Harry Hampton? Even though he flirted with her, she wasn't foolish enough to think that he didn't flirt with every woman. Nothing was ever going to come of it. He'd never be interested in someone like her. And even if he were, she'd never permit anything to happen between them. *Blimey*, she thought. She could just imagine the gossip it would cause. Tongues would wag right across the borough. She'd put herself in an impossible situation and she had to get her daft feelings into check, once and for all.

7

On Wednesday morning, Harry sat at the kitchen table with his very tired-looking family. Even Errol was home for breakfast, which was a rarity these days. Harry had hoped that the presence of their son would have put Carmen in a better mood but she looked as miserable as ever.

'I've hardly slept. I don't know how I'm going to keep me eyes open at work today,' Cheryl moaned.

'Don't worry, sweetheart, everyone will be in the same boat,' Harry assured his daughter.

'The all-clear went off at four-thirty this morning, it's ridiculous. Why do they attack at night, Dad?'

'Visibility. They use the dark to hide in. Then they're more likely to get past our air defences in Kent, straight up the Thames Estuary and into London.'

Carmen leaned over his shoulder and spooned scrambled eggs from a pan onto his plate. 'Thanks, love,' Harry said. Picking up his knife and fork, he turned to his son. 'Are you around today?'

'Dunno. I could be, I suppose,' Errol answered moodily.

'Good. I've got a little job for you. Meet me in the Battersea Tavern at lunchtime.'

Carmen huffed, making Harry wonder what was wrong with her. He'd assumed her sour face was due to being exhausted after four nights of air raids. Now he suspected that there was more to it. But he wouldn't challenge her now, not in front of the kids. Especially as it made a nice change for them all to be having breakfast together.

'Errol, me and Yvonne are going to the dance on Saturday afternoon, the one up at the Town Hall. Are you going?' Cheryl asked her brother.

'No, not my thing.'

'How do you know, if you've never been before?'

'I know. Anyway, I'm busy.'

'Oh yeah, doing what?'

'None of your business, missy.'

'Go with your sister,' Carmen snapped as she pulled out a seat at the table and sat down in front of an empty plate.

'But I'm busy,' Errol argued.

'Then make yourself un-busy. I want you at that dance to keep an eye on her.'

Cheryl looked outraged. 'I don't need anyone to keep an eye on me, thank you very much!' she exclaimed.

'Maybe not, but your brother can keep an eye on any soldiers who think that they can take advantage of you.'

'I'm not a child!'

'Mum's right,' Errol said. 'I'll be there.'

'Great, but that's not why I wanted you to come.'

'Why, then?'

'I dunno. Maybe you could have a dance with Yvonne?' Cheryl asked sheepishly.

Errol guffawed and answered, 'I ain't desperate.'

'Don't be mean,' Carmen said. 'Yvonne's a lovely young lady.'

'You could do worse,' Harry added.

'He has,' Cheryl said sarcastically, 'Stephanie Reynolds.'

'Who? Did you say Stephanie Reynolds?' Carmen asked.

Harry saw Errol look at his sister with daggers in his eyes. But Cheryl ignored his glare and nodded at her mum.

'You've got to be kidding me!' Carmen screeched. She scraped her seat back and went to the sink, banging the cutlery and crockery on the side. 'That girl is nothing more than a common whore. How could you, Errol? You can do so much better than Stephanie Reynolds.'

'I'm not marrying the girl, Mum. I like her, she's fun, that's all.'

'No, you most certainly are not marrying her, ever! I won't have that tart as a daughter-in-law! Don't you dare get her in the family way. Oh my Gawd, that's the last thing I need. Stephanie Reynolds being the mother to my firstborn grand-child. I won't have it, Errol, I'm warning you. Keep it in your trousers!'

Harry rolled his eyes at his son who discreetly smiled at him. Even Cheryl looked bemused at her mother's outburst.

Carmen spun back round from the sink, her eyes darting across each of them. 'I know what you're all thinking and you can take the micky out of me as much as you like, but am I the only one who cares about this family's reputation? Eh?'

'No, love, come and sit down. Cheryl, pour your mother a cuppa.'

'Don't patronise me, Harry. I've got Errol knocking about with a tart. Cheryl drinking in a pub. And you're as bad, carting that Winnie Berry about in your sidecar. Have you thought about how that looks?'

So that was it. Carmen had seen him give Winnie a lift and now she had her knickers in a twist about it. Harry had known something was bothering his wife but he hadn't expected her to be upset over Winnie. Or maybe his wife had an inkling that he had feelings for the woman. 'Her daughter is in hospital, lucky to be alive. I picked her up and dropped her off at home, that's all. There's nothing to be made of that.'

'You know full well that Jan isn't Winnie's *real* daughter and it's something they've made up between themselves. Tell me, Harry, if you've got nothing to hide, why didn't you mention to me that you'd given Winnie a lift? Or is there more to it? I mean, you spend more time in her pub than you do at home!'

'For Christ's sake, woman, do I have to run every tiny detail of my day past you? I've told you so many times already, I'm in the pub selling me gear.'

Cheryl got up from the table, looking annoyed. 'I'm going to work,' she barked and then stamped out of the kitchen. Errol followed her.

'See – see what you've done,' Harry said, gesticulating towards the kitchen door. Once again, his wife had started an argument in front of the kids and ruined a pleasant morning. He pushed his plate away. Carmen's jealous accusations had put him off his food.

'What *I've* done? You're the one who's ferrying that fat old cow around behind my back. I had to hear about it from the woman in the haberdashery shop. She made me feel two inches tall. So don't you blame me for this.'

Harry drew in a long, deep breath. He knew there was no

point in rising to Carmen's scathing remarks about Winnie. 'I've got to go to work, sweetheart, but rest assured, I'm not hiding anything from you and there's nothing going on with me and Winnie. I'll see you this evening.' He went to place a light kiss on Carmen's tight lips but she turned her face so he pecked her cheek instead.

Outside, the morning was bright and pleasant and Harry was pleased to be away from the hostility in the kitchen. Carmen had recently moaned about being left stuck indoors by herself all day but she did nothing to make him feel that he wanted to rush home to her. In fact, Harry realised with a saddened heart, he looked forward to seeing Winnie more than he did his wife. He enjoyed her company. She was always jolly and had a kind heart. The complete opposite to Carmen, who could never find a nice word to say about anyone. He checked his watch. Winnie wouldn't have left for the hospital yet. She'd said she didn't want a lift but Harry would insist. He pulled on his helmet and set off towards the Battersea Tavern with a smile on his face. At least Winnie would offer him a warm welcome and a cup of tea without a tongue-lashing.

Cheryl hadn't wanted to stay at home and listen to her parents arguing again. She left the house and arrived at the factory early but was disappointed to see Ada waiting outside the gates. The woman had a scarf round her head, tied under her double chin, and a faded wool coat that barely stretched across her ample chest. In contrast, Cheryl had thrown on her smart fur-trimmed coat and matching hat. She was fully aware that she was overdressed compared to the other women in the factory but she didn't care. She liked nice clothes and, as her mum had said on many occasions, they didn't have to drop their standards to match those of the neighbours.

Cheryl was in no mood for any of Ada's snide remarks today and also lacked the energy to fight back. But as she approached the woman, she braced herself, ready for whatever Ada had to throw at her.

'You're keen, or did you piss your bed?' Ada asked and then drew on her cigarette.

'I could ask you the same question but I won't because I couldn't care less.'

'Suits me. Let's be honest. You Hamptons have never cared about anyone other than yourselves.'

'We look after our own. There's nothing wrong with that.'

'Ha, don't make me laugh, Cheryl. You don't look after your own at all. What about your gran over in Balham? None of you lot have been near her in years. Is that your idea of looking after your own?'

Cheryl stared blankly at Ada, her mind turning. What was the woman on about? As far as Cheryl knew, all her grandparents were dead. Ada must be mistaken; it was the only explanation.

'Got nothing to say for yourself now? No, I thought not. Your lot should be ashamed of yourselves, leaving that poor old woman to fend for herself. My sister lives a few doors down from her and does more for your gran than her own family does!'

'You don't know what you're talking about. My grandparents died years ago.'

'They might as well have, for all the attention you give them. But Edie Hampton is very much alive, no thanks to you and yours.'

For once, Cheryl was left speechless. She felt the urge to run back home and ask her mum and dad if what Ada had said was true. But someone tapped her on the shoulder and she turned to see Yvonne.

'Morning, Cheryl, you're early.'

Cheryl linked her arm through her friend's and pulled her along the street and out of Ada's earshot. She glanced over her shoulder to see Ada looking very smug as she threw her cigarette to the ground.

'Are you all right?' Yvonne asked.

'Yeah, yeah, I'm fine. But Ada said something a bit strange.'

'You know you shouldn't take any notice of anything she says.'

'Yeah, I know, but this was different. She was on about my gran who lives in Balham.'

'I thought all your grandparents were dead?'

'So did I but now I'm not so sure.'

'You'll have to ask your mum. She'll know.'

'Yes, but why would my mum and dad have told me that my gran was dead if she isn't?'

'I don't know, that's a bit weird. It's probably Ada just trying to cause problems as usual.'

'Hmm, maybe,' Cheryl said wistfully. 'Or maybe she was telling the truth. But either way, I'm going to get to the bottom of it.'

The morning flew by for Lucy. She happily served customers, filled shelves, wiped down tables and emptied ashtrays but her mind was elsewhere. She had something to look forward to. She'd arranged to meet David and was excited about seeing him again. Just as she'd first thought, he'd been nothing like how Winnie, Rachel and Hilda had described him. In fact, Lucy had found him to be thoroughly charming and every inch the gentleman. As far as she could see, David had been unfairly branded by his mother and her friends as a liar and a thief and she was glad that she hadn't allowed the witches' opinion of him to sway her own.

'Psst,' Rachel hissed, her head poking through the door from the passageway. 'The kettle's on. Fancy a cuppa once you've locked up? I've made some rock cakes too.'

Lucy had to think on her feet if she was going to get out of the invitation. 'Erm – thanks, but I've got to pop over to see my mum. She's had a fall and wants me to help her with some shopping,' she lied.

'Just a quick one? I'm bored stiff up there and Martha will be asleep for a good hour.'

'I really shouldn't. My mum is expecting me.'

Rachel sighed. 'I wish I could come with you and give you a hand with the shopping but I dare not leave the place in case I bump into David. Has anyone mentioned seeing him?'

'No, not a dickie bird.'

'Maybe he's gone back to whatever rock he crawled out from under. Perhaps I could come with you? Martha could do with the fresh air and she'll sleep in the pram.'

Lucy could feel her pulse quicken. 'No, I don't think you should risk it, not just yet. You'd be really upset if you bumped into him. And what about Martha? You don't want her to see you upset.'

'Yeah, I suppose you're right. But I can't hide away forever. Oh well. Winnie will be back soon. She'll cheer me up.'

'I could take Martha out with me? Like you said, she could do with the fresh air.'

'Oh, thanks, but I don't know.'

'It's no bother, I'd like to.'

'She hasn't been away from me and what if she wants a feed?'

'It's fine, I understand. Perhaps next time? You could get a bottle ready and it'll give you more time to get used to the idea. You never know, you might enjoy the break for a couple of hours.'

'That's a smashing idea, thanks, Lucy. I'll think about it.'

Rachel slipped away back upstairs and Lucy puffed out a long breath of relief. That had been a close call but she'd managed to get away with it. Though she did question why she was sneaking around behind Rachel's and Winnie's backs. After all, she was a grown woman and could make her own decisions. And who she saw was nothing to do with the *witches*. Though sneaking around might not be a bad thing at the moment, especially if she could get Martha away from Rachel for a while. She was sure that David would love to see his daughter and bringing her along would earn Lucy good favour with him.

Moments later, Winnie bustled in looking very rosy-cheeked. She patted the scarf covering her head as she walked towards the bar, chuckling, with Harry beside her.

'You're looking happy. I take it Jan is on the mend?' Lucy asked.

'Better than that. She'll be discharged tomorrow and she's engaged! Terry proposed last night and she accepted. I'm chuffed to bits, I really am!'

'Aw, that's smashing.'

'It is. Are you all right down here? I just want to nip upstairs and tell Rachel the happy news.'

'Yes, I'm fine.'

'Thanks, love. And get Harry a drink, on the house.'

As Lucy fetched a bottle of ale for Harry, she saw the door open again and Harry's son amble in. Errol had a mysterious air about him and she thought he was just as attractive as David. But he didn't have David's charm and seemed to lack a sense of humour. Their eyes locked as he came towards the bar but Lucy decided that of the two men, though Errol dressed immaculately, she'd chosen well in picking David. Especially as Errol still lived with his parents and didn't have a steady job. He had little to offer. Unlike David, who had his own place in Richmond and worked for the electric board. David had prospects and could offer her the life she dreamed of – a home away from stinking Battersea with a man who could provide for her and the children she desperately wanted.

8

In Battersea Park, Lucy sat on a blanket on the ground next to the boating lake. When she'd suggested that they meet in the park, she'd thought that David had been very thoughtful to have brought the blanket and some stale bread to feed the geese. 'I should go soon,' she said reluctantly. She looked across the lake and then back at David, hoping with anticipation that he would kiss her.

'It is getting a bit chilly,' he said and reached for her hand.

'I've had a lovely couple of hours. And I'm hoping to bring Martha with me next time.'

'Really? Rachel will allow her to see me?'

'Oh, no, sorry, nothing like that. But she did say that I could take her out for a walk. There's no need for Rachel to know that I'll be bringing Martha to see you.'

'You devious little minx,' David said with a wicked smile. 'You'd do that for me?'

'Yes, of course I would. Martha is your child; you've every right to see her.'

'Yeah, but they won't see it like that. I bet they think I've got no rights because I left before she was born. But it wasn't like that, like they say. There was a lot more to it.'

Lucy was dying to know David's reasons but said sweetly, 'It's all right, you don't have to explain anything to me. I know you're not a bad man.'

'Thanks, but I'll tell you what happened. If you're going to be my girl, then you should know the truth.'

His girl! Lucy could have squealed with delight but she kept her reactions in check. 'OK,' she answered calmly.

'See, the thing is, I didn't know for sure if Rachel was pregnant. I mean, she wasn't my girl or anything like that. She was seeing this other bloke, Arnold. He dumped her and she got upset, drowned her sorrows with booze, or so I'm told. I was asleep upstairs and had no idea what was going on, till Rachel sneaked into my bed. I didn't realise that she was three sheets gone to the wind and, well, you know, one thing led to another. The next thing I know, I heard she had a bun in the oven but I didn't know if the baby was mine or Arnold's. Let's face it, Rachel is a nice girl but she's got the morals of an alley cat. I didn't want to be lumbered married to her. I know that sounds harsh but it's the truth.'

Lucy looked into his eyes and believed every word. 'I suppose you had to steal some money so that you could run off?'

'I wasn't running away from Rachel and the baby. It was the army, Lucy. I'd signed up but I knew I'd be useless on a battlefield. I might just as well have signed me own death warrant. I couldn't face it. I must sound like such a coward but I'm just not made for fighting. And yeah, I needed the money. I'd been off work sick for months with a bad back so I was skint. I couldn't ask me mum for money. She'd just *adopted* Jan, a grown woman. It was ridiculous. Me mum had no time for me anymore. She brought home a complete stranger and told me that the woman was my sister. I mean, come on, it was obvious that she wasn't. But they carried on like long-lost family and I got ousted out. In fact, I'm pretty sure that Jan was pinching money from me mum and blaming me! What did I need money for, eh? I was laid up in bed, I couldn't go anywhere or do anything. So once I was better and when I had the chance to get away, I did. I hated taking the money and still feel terrible about it.'

'Oh, David, what a rotten time for you. Have you told your mum all that you've told me?'

'Yeah, but she won't forgive me. I can't say I blame her, really. Stealing the pub's takings was wrong; I should never have done it.'

'But you only did it because you was scared of being sent to war. She shouldn't blame you for that. I would have been scared too and maybe done the same as you. Your mum is a hard woman.'

'Yeah, she is. Why do you think my dad did a runner, eh? She was mean to him an' all. My dad was a good man. I haven't seen him for ages; he could be dead, for all I know. I miss him, and it's all because of my mother.'

'Blimey, she comes across so nice. I'll watch myself around her from now on.'

'Yeah, I would. You get my mum, Rachel and Hilda to-gether – well, it's not a good combination.'

Lucy lowered her eyes and smirked. 'I call them *the witches*,' she giggled.

'You ain't wrong there!'

She felt his finger under her chin and he gently lifted her head. As she gazed into his eyes, his face came towards her and she knew she was going to receive that long-awaited kiss. His mouth felt warm and gentle on her lips. When he pulled away, Lucy was left tingling and wanting more. She swallowed hard. 'I really should get going,' she whispered.

'I'll walk you out of the park but I don't think I should come to the pub.'

'Are you staying in Battersea?'

'Yes, but I don't know for how much longer. I came back to make amends with my mum but she doesn't want to know. There wasn't much for me to stay here for till I met you.'

Lucy could feel her cheeks flush. It seemed that David was just as smitten with her as she was with him. 'Don't you have to get back to work?' she asked.

'Yes, I will, soon. Can we meet tomorrow? Maybe you could bring Martha?'

'I'd like that,' Lucy answered.

She didn't want to go back to the pub and act nicely to Winnie and Rachel. They had no idea how much they'd hurt David or maybe they just didn't care. Either way, she decided she didn't like them. David deserved better and Lucy would do all she could to make him happy. After all, isn't that what a good wife was supposed to do?

Cheryl had managed to avoid Ada all day but she couldn't stop thinking about what the woman had told her. Could she really have a gran living just up the road in Balham? And if her name was Edie Hampton, then it followed that Edie was her father's mother.

There had been excited chatter all day amongst the women on her work bench. Carol and Anne were really looking forward to the dance on Saturday and Yvonne seemed really enthusiastic about it now too. Cheryl had tried to join in but the thought of her gran living alone and abandoned by her family overshadowed everything.

'It's nearly clocking-off time. Anne and Carol are going to the Battersea Tavern. Shall we join them?' Yvonne asked.

'No, thanks. You go. I want to get home and ask my mum about my gran,' Cheryl whispered.

Twenty minutes later, Cheryl charged through her front door and straight into the kitchen where her mum was preparing dinner. 'I need to talk to you,' Cheryl blurted breathlessly.

Her mum turned around from the stove and wiped her hands on the front of her apron. 'I'm in the middle of something, you can see that. And go and take your coat off, you're indoors, my kitchen isn't a yard.'

Cheryl marched from the kitchen, removed her coat, then threw it over the bannisters before rushing back into the steamy room.

Her mum was pouring a cup of tea. 'Here you go. I expect you're gasping.'

'Thanks. Mum, can you sit down with me for a minute, please?'

'I told you, I'm busy. I'm just about to mash the spuds.'

'Mum, please, this is important. Just leave them for a while.'

Her mother huffed as she turned off the gas under the pot of potatoes. She sat opposite Cheryl at the table with her hands intertwined in front of her. 'What's this all about?' she asked.

Cheryl looked her mother straight in the eye. 'Is my gran alive and does she live in Balham?'

Her mother quickly stood up and went back to the stove, but not before Cheryl had seen her face pale.

'Well, is she?' Cheryl pushed.

'No, don't be daft. Your gran died years ago, before you was born.'

'So why did Ada at work tell me that Edie Hampton, my gran, lives on the same street as her sister?'

'I don't know. The woman has a big mouth and spouts a load of rubbish. You should know better than to listen to the likes of her!'

Cheryl drummed her fingers on the table. She didn't believe her mother. But she knew there was no point in pursuing it. Instead, she sipped on her cup of tea, her mind turning. If she couldn't prise the truth from her mother, perhaps she'd have better luck with her father. If not, as a last resort, she'd bite the bullet and ask Ada where her sister lived and go and see Edie Hampton for herself.

Winnie whistled as she worked and when she wasn't whistling, she was beaming with delight. Just a couple of days ago she'd feared that Jan was dead but now her daughter was due out of hospital and was going to marry Terry Card. She thought Terry was a good lad and she couldn't be happier about welcoming him into the family. But there was still a blot on her landscape – David was in Battersea.

'Congratulations to the happy couple,' Bill said and raised his glass to Winnie.

'Oh, Bill, I'm thrilled, I really am. And Terry has already said that they will hold the wedding celebrations in here. I can't wait. I'm going to throw them the best party Battersea has ever seen.'

'When are they tying the knot?'

'I'm not sure, but it'll be sooner rather than later. Terry has got it in his head that's he's going to jack his job in at the baker's and go and sign up. I wish he wouldn't but there's no talking to him about it.'

'He's a young man, Winnie, it's only natural that he'd want to do his bit.'

'I suppose so, but I can't stand to think of anything happening to him and my Jan being left a widow.'

'You can't think like that. Now, stop being so maudlin and fill me glass up.'

'Please,' Winnie reminded Bill.

'Please,' Bill parroted.

As Winnie handed Bill his refilled glass, the door opened and she was happy to see a few girls come in from the local factory. They hadn't been in for a while. She thought they brightened the place up and made her male customers watch their Ps and Qs. 'Hello, ladies. What can I get you?' she asked.

'Just three ginger beers, please,' Carol answered.

'Go and sit down, I'll send them over.' Winnie admired the women's spirit. They'd taken on the roles of a man's job and were willing to drink in a pub without a snug or without being accompanied by a bloke. She thought it was about time that women had more freedom and control over their lives, though she'd heard that they were receiving less pay than a man would get for doing the same job.

The women went over to a corner table next to the table where Harry usually sat. Anne, the tallest, led the way. She had striking red hair and bright green eyes. Winnie assumed she was of Irish origin. In contrast, Carol, the shortest girl, had dark blonde hair and blue eyes. She was a pretty girl but she carried herself awkwardly, probably due to the size of her huge chest. And then there was Yvonne. A shy young lady and not blessed with the good looks of her friends.

'Lucy, take these over to the ladies in the corner, please,' Winnie said, indicating some bottles and glasses on a tray.

Lucy looked past Winnie and pulled a face of disgust. 'Do I have to? I can't stand Carol and Anne.'

'Yes, you do. When you're behind my bar, you put your differences aside and get on with your job.'

'But, Winnie, they don't like me either,' Lucy moaned.

'Oh, for Gawd's sake,' Winnie snapped and tutted. She had no patience for this. 'Collect some glasses, then. But you need to pull your socks up, young lady!'

Winnie carried the tray over and couldn't wait to tell the women about Jan and Terry. As she approached, she noticed they were looking at Lucy scathingly and whispering amongst themselves. She placed the tray on the table and cleared her throat, then leaned in towards them. 'I know you and Lucy don't get on, but I'll thank you to be polite in my pub and I won't accept any catty remarks. Is that clear?'

They all nodded simultaneously. It was Carol who spoke. 'A word of warning, Mrs Berry. Watch her, especially around the men.'

'What's that supposed to mean?' Winnie asked quietly.

'I shouldn't say but I think you deserve to know. She's not right in the head. She's obsessed with getting married. She scares blokes off.'

'There's nothing wrong with a young lady wanting to settle down,' Winnie said in Lucy's defence.

'No, Mrs Berry, you don't understand. I mean *really*

obsessed. It's weird. She sets her eyes on a fella and then follows him around everywhere. She latched on to my neighbour's brother. It caused no end of problems. That's why me and Lucy are no longer friends.'

'What sort of problems?' Winnie probed, beginning to feel slightly concerned.

'Well, me and Lucy used to pop round to my neighbour's house a few times a week. Then, on the quiet, my neighbour said her brother, Gerry, started noticing that things were *disappearing* from his room. Little things like his comb and his lighter. Then Lucy started turning up at Gerry's work and wouldn't take a hint. In the end, Gerry told her to leave him alone. That's when Lucy turned nasty. She wrote to his boss and told him that Gerry had attacked her in Battersea Park, by the boating lake. He nearly lost his job over it. She got parcels sent to Gerry's mum of her clothes, ripped and muddied, with notes, saying Gerry had done it. She even followed him and his girlfriend into the cinema and started screaming about what he'd done. None of it was true. Luckily, Gerry could prove it. So, all I'm saying is, watch her.'

Winnie glanced over at Lucy, her eyes narrowing. Lucy was leaning against the back counter and chewing her nails nervously. Winnie wondered if what Carol had said held any truth. She'd seen no sign of Lucy *latching* on to any of her customers, but then with Jan being in hospital, Winnie hadn't been around much. The trouble with gossip was that it always got twisted and distorted as it spread around and Winnie thought that this could be the case here. After all, she didn't know this Gerry. Maybe there was more to it than Carol had said. Perhaps he had attacked Lucy and she was the victim here. Whatever the case, Winnie was willing to give Lucy a fair chance. The girl had done no wrong in her eyes and worked hard. But, none the less, she'd keep a closer eye on her from now on, just in case.

As soon as Harry walked into the Battersea Tavern, he spotted his daughter's friends sitting at the table next to his customary spot. He wondered where Cheryl was. It was unusual to see Yvonne in the pub without Cheryl. Winnie was there too, having a chat with Carol.

'Hello, ladies,' he greeted them, doffing his trilby hat.

'Hello, Mr Hampton,' the girls chirped and Winnie offered her usual friendly smile.

Harry ached to hold Winnie in his arms and kiss her big smile but he had to remain composed, especially in front of Cheryl's friends. 'My Cheryl not with you?' he asked the girls.

'No, Mr Hampton, she went straight home after work,' Yvonne answered.

'Your usual, Harry?' Winnie asked.

'Yes, please, sweetheart. Do you girls want a drink?'

'No, thanks, Mr Hampton, we're fine.'

'I'll have one,' Cheryl said.

Harry turned around to see his daughter had come in and noticed that she looked unusually sombre. 'Hello, sweetheart. Everything all right at home?'

'Yeah, but Mum won't be happy that we're not home for tea. She was dishing up as I left.'

'Couldn't you have had your dinner before coming out?'

'No, I'd like a word with you.'

'All right. This sounds serious. Sit down, I'll get us a drink.'

'No, not here, in private,' Cheryl said.

Harry looked around. The bar was quite busy; he couldn't

see a spot that would be very private. 'Do you want to have a chat outside?'

'You can go through to my back kitchen, if you like?' Winnie offered.

'Thanks, Winnie,' Harry said and he signed to Cheryl to follow him. Something wasn't right with his daughter; she was acting out of character and his heart raced as a tirade of awful scenarios flashed through his mind. Christ, he hoped she hadn't got herself in the family way. Carmen would do her nut!

He pulled out a seat at the small kitchen table as he asked, 'Now, what's this all about?'

Cheryl's face was grave. 'Is my gran living in Balham?'

Harry baulked. Of all the things that he had imagined that could be wrong with Cheryl, he hadn't expected this. She'd been so direct with her question, it caught Harry off guard and he wasn't sure how to answer her. 'Erm … sweetheart, what makes you – er – think that?' he asked, stumbling over his words.

'Ada at work told me that her sister lives near to my gran, Edie Hampton. Is it true? Is your mum alive?'

Harry gulped. He wasn't sure how to get out of this. He could feel his brow beginning to perspire. If he told his daughter the truth, Carmen's family history would come out and he knew his wife would be furious. And that was only the half of it. His mother knew too much about things that Harry hoped would never come to light.

'It *is* true, isn't it? I knew it! Why have you lied to me all these years? How could you leave your own mother alone to look after herself? Oh, Dad, what's going on?'

Harry looked down at his lap, suddenly feeling very

ashamed. No matter how he tried to explain the situation, it was going to look bad. 'It's a long story, darling, and all in the past. It's best left there.'

'No, Dad, it's not in the past, is it? My gran is alive. I've never even met her. What did she do that was so awful as to warrant being abandoned by her own family?'

The truth was, Harry's mother *hadn't* done anything that bad. He'd turned his back on her and had cut her out of his life to save himself from looking bad. It had been so many years ago that he hardly thought about her anymore – not till now. The shame that washed over him was also mixed with guilt. She'd been a good mum in many ways and had only been trying to do the right thing.

Cheryl's voice interrupted his thoughts. 'Please, Dad, tell me what happened?'

Harry looked into his daughter's pleading eyes and knew that he was about to disappoint her. 'It was when I met your mother,' he said. 'My mum didn't approve of Carmen. She tried to stop me from seeing her.'

'You chose my mum over your mum?'

'Yeah, I did. I loved your mother with all me heart. I wouldn't have let anyone come in between us.'

'That's all well and good, Dad, but surely once you was married and had us, my gran would have come round?'

Harry sighed deeply. 'There's more to it than that, sweetheart. You know the truth now, let's just leave it there, eh?'

'But that's your mother! She's never done anything to hurt me. You might want to pretend that she doesn't exist but I won't. I'm going to see her.'

Before Harry could discourage his daughter, she stamped

out of the kitchen. He followed her out and found her sitting with her friends, but she made a point of ignoring him.

Winnie placed a bottle and glass on his table. 'Everything all right?' she asked discreetly.

Harry shrugged. 'Family stuff,' he said and rolled his eyes. If Cheryl saw her gran, she would discover Carmen's heritage and a lot more besides. He knew how determined Cheryl could be and couldn't see how he could dissuade her from visiting his mother. If truth be told, he knew that he should see the old girl too. She'd be getting on now. If he didn't act soon, it might be too late. But he couldn't face her, not ever.

Cheryl's voice carried over. Harry could hear she was talking about the dance on Saturday. 'Sorry to interrupt, ladies,' he said, 'but haven't you heard? The dance has been cancelled on account of the air raids.'

'Oh, no, we were really looking forward to it,' Cheryl groaned. 'Blinkin' Hitler! It's not fair.'

'What dance is this?' Winnie asked.

'At the Town Hall. We were all going to wear our best dresses and try to enjoy ourselves for a few hours.'

'I tell you what, how about we have a big party here for Terry and Jan's engagement?'

'That would be smashing, Mrs Berry,' the young women chorused.

'We could all make something to bring, you know, sandwiches and stuff,' Carol offered.

'No need, love, I'll sort out the food. You just bring yourselves along. Oh, it'll be lovely,' Winnie said excitedly and clapped her hands together.

Harry smiled at the girls' delighted faces though, inside, he was in turmoil. It was going to be awkward and there would be an awful atmosphere in the Anderson shelter if they all had to cram into it again tonight. Much had been left unspoken. Should he tell Cheryl about Carmen before she heard it from her gran? But then there was still the other issue, the one that Harry had pushed from his mind. A stab of guilt pierced his heart as the memories came flooding back. Cheryl and Errol would never understand what he and Carmen had done. He couldn't allow his mother to expose the truth. But should he visit her? Would she even want to see him? Every question in his head led to the same answer – he'd never have the nerve to knock on his mother's door. It was inevitable that Cheryl would discover the truth, and when she did, Harry knew that Carmen was going to be impossible to live with.

He walked back to the bar with a heavy heart and tense shoulders.

'Kids, eh,' Winnie said. 'I don't know what family problems you've got going on, but I've got a few of my own.'

'I hope Brian's not bothering you. You've no need to be worried about him anymore, Winnie. If he's getting to you, just give me the nod, I'll pay him a visit.'

'No, no, nothing like that. As long as Brian gets paid, he's no bother. It's David. I suppose you've heard he's back in Battersea.'

'Yes, I have.'

'With everything that's been going on with Jan, I've not been able to think straight. But you know what David's like. Trouble follows him.'

'Has he been to see you?'

'Yeah, but I threw him out. It's horrible, Harry. You're a father, you know what it's like. I love the boy but he's a bad 'un, just like his father.'

Harry knew *exactly* how Winnie felt. 'Yeah, I know what you mean. Look at Errol. He's not a lad to be proud of.'

'But you love him all the same.'

'I don't know. If I'm honest, I don't feel the same about him as I do my Cheryl.'

'Maybe because he's a lad and she's a girl.'

'Hmm, maybe. But it feels natural with Cheryl.'

'And it doesn't with Errol?'

'No, not at all. I'm not sure that I even like him.'

'He's a difficult bloke to like.'

'Not 'alf! Between you and me, I wonder if he really is my son.'

Winnie looked back at him, her eyes wide, and Harry realised that he'd revealed too much. 'Forget I said that.'

'Do you think that Carmen had an affair?' Winnie asked.

'No, I know she didn't. But, it's complicated and a long story that happened years ago. I shouldn't have said anything.'

'But you did. Listen, Harry, if ever you want to talk, you know I'll always give you my ear.'

'Yeah, thanks, Winnie. And likewise. We go back a long time, you and me. You're a good friend,' he said with a smile. But Harry wanted more than just Winnie's friendship. Though he could never tell her how he really felt. It was just another secret that he had to harbour.

9

When Cheryl arrived home from the pub, she went straight upstairs to her bedroom and closed the door behind her. She sat on her bed, disgusted with her parents. They had lied to her for her whole life. She wondered what else they were hiding.

'Cheryl, Cheryl,' her mother's voice sounded from the bottom of the stairs.

Cheryl ignored her. She couldn't bring herself to answer. Just a couple of hours earlier, she had asked her mum about her gran only to be fed more untruths. At least her father had been honest when pressed, though he hadn't divulged everything. Her jaw clenched in anger. *Wait till Errol hears about this*, she thought, desperate to speak to her brother.

'Cheryl, your dinner is in the oven. It'll be ruined by now.'

'Go away,' Cheryl hissed under her breath. She was too uptight to eat and didn't want to have to even look at her mother.

'CHERYL! Did you hear me?'

Cheryl leapt from the bed and pulled open the door. 'Yes, I heard you. I'm not hungry,' she shouted back and slammed the door closed again.

Then she heard her mother pounding up the stairs and Cheryl's heart sank. She knew her mother was coming for her.

Carmen didn't knock on the door. She pushed it open forcibly. She glared at Cheryl and growled, 'Don't take that tone with me. Get downstairs now and eat your dinner. If I've been good enough to cook it, you can bloody well eat it.'

Cheryl turned away from her mum's angry eyes and she stared towards her bedroom window. 'I said, I'm not hungry,' she seethed.

'Been stuffing your face at the pub, have you? Well, that's choice, that is. You knew full well that I was dishing up your tea.'

Cheryl didn't answer, afraid that if she opened her mouth, she'd say something that she would regret.

'You're so ungrateful. I don't know why I bother!'

Thankfully, her mother left in a flurry of fury, slamming the door and sounding as if she were deliberately banging down the stairs as loudly as she could. Cheryl sighed with relief. She didn't want a confrontation about her gran with her mother. If her parents wouldn't tell her the full story, she'd find out for herself, directly from the horse's mouth. Even if that meant asking Ada for the address.

In the quietness of her room, as she sat and imagined what her gran was like, she heard a distant hum approaching and was suddenly filled with a foreboding feeling of dread. Instantly she knew that the Luftwaffe were returning. Fear coursed through her. She'd seen the shocking images in the newspapers of the East End, parts of it almost flattened by bombs. She'd heard that there had been a few local hits too. Moaning Minnie sprang into life, the wailing warning noise screeching out. The planes were closer now and Cheryl's heart hammered in time with the sound of the anti-aircraft fire. Ack-ack guns shot their defensive ammunition skyward as Spitfires attacked the oncoming German bombers and fighter planes. She covered her ears with her hands, trying to block out the terrifying sounds.

Her bedroom door flew open again and her mother, ashen-faced, pulled on Cheryl's arm.

'Don't just sit there! Come on, down to the shelter.'

Cheryl didn't put up any resistance and allowed her mother to drag her down the stairs, through the kitchen and out of the back door. The air outside felt damp. She looked up to see searchlights overhead, scanning the dark sky, planes silhouetted against the black backdrop of the clouds.

Her mother had released her grip and pulled on the shelter door. 'Hurry up,' she snapped as she entered the corrugated-iron shelter.

Cheryl dreaded the thought of getting inside the Anderson, and even more so, the thought of being in such close proximity to her mother. She looked back for her father. He must still be in the pub where she'd left him cutting a deal with a man from the factory where she worked.

'Cheryl, don't just stand there!' her mother shouted.

Her mum's urgent voice spurred her into action and Cheryl ran towards the shelter. As she settled down on a camp bed, pulling a blanket over her legs, her mum spoke again.

'I don't know what's got into you. I hope you've not been drinking?'

'No,' Cheryl managed to answer, giving her mum a side-ways glance.

Her mum lit a gas lamp and busied herself checking

their supplies. 'Gawd knows where your father is. Still in the bleedin' pub, no doubt. I hope he gets his backside here soon.'

As her mother finished her sentence, the Anderson door opened and her father stuck his head inside. 'Here we go again,' he said cheerily, which Cheryl found out of context, given that there were planes engaged in a dogfight directly overhead. They didn't only have the bombs landing on them to worry about. Planes being shot down, or parts of planes that had exploded in the sky, could come falling down too.

Cheryl turned over on the camp bed to face the wall. She watched a spider scurry up the iron sheeting and back to its web. Her mind wandered back to thoughts of her gran. She wondered if the woman was safe. Or was she scared? She hoped not. Again, anger bubbled within as she realised that her parents probably hadn't considered how Edie Hampton was faring in these frightening times.

She heard her mum talking to her dad. 'Oh no, I've left the oven on with your dinner in it.'

'Don't worry, I'll go and turn it off.'

'No, Harry, you can't go out there.'

'It's fine. I won't be a tick.'

Cheryl felt the cold air rush in as her father left the shelter. She held her breath, listening for every sound, praying that nothing would fall on their house. Just a minute later, he returned, chuckling to himself.

'This looks tasty,' he said.

'It's dried up. Ruined.'

'No, it's fine. Here, Cheryl, your dinner.'

Cheryl didn't want to turn around and look at her parents. Instead, she squeezed her eyes shut and pretended to be asleep.

'Cheryl, your dinner,' her father repeated.

'She's in one of her moods. Leave her be. She can go hungry,' her mother said.

Cheryl felt like she'd been lying on the camp bed for hours. She'd heard the rustle of a newspaper and her mother's knitting needles clicking. Now all she could hear was her father's soft snoring, the faraway sound of the Luftwaffe and RAF fighting and the low thud of bombs dropping. Nothing vibrated around them. The explosions must be a long way off. It offered Cheryl some peace of mind but she couldn't sleep. Images of a petrified old lady flooded her mind. No matter what the rest of the night brought, Cheryl would travel to Balham tomorrow and finally meet her gran.

Harry was sure that Cheryl was asleep but he couldn't be sure. He pulled a small notepad from his jacket pocket, licked the end of his pencil, and scribbled a note to Carmen: *Cheryl asked about my mother. She knows she's alive.* He offered the note to his wife whilst holding his finger over his lips to tell her to be quiet.

Carmen put her knitting on her lap and took the note. She read it, then handed it back, her face expressionless.

Harry quickly scribbled again. *I think she will go and see her.*

After Carmen read this, she reached out for the pencil. *You'll have to make sure that she doesn't.*

How? Harry wrote back.

I don't know. You shouldn't have told her that she's alive. You had better sort this out! Carmen replied.

Harry slumped into the deckchair. It was clear that Carmen was putting the blame on him and wasn't going to help resolve the uncomfortable situation. But he had no idea how he was going to prevent Cheryl from seeing his mother. After all, Cheryl was a grown woman, so he could hardly stop her by threatening to smack the back of her legs. He knew that he'd have to come up with something inventive before all hell broke loose and a family feud ensued.

Lucy sat in the cellar and looked at the words in her book but they floated in front of her eyes and wouldn't sink in. Her mind was elsewhere – on David. She'd spent a pleasant couple of hours with him earlier and had managed to persuade Rachel to allow her to take Martha out. Of course, Rachel had no idea that Lucy was introducing Martha to David. Had Rachel known, she would never have allowed it.

Lucy had been surprised at David's nonchalant attitude towards his daughter. She'd expected him to be gushy and to shower Martha with affection. Instead, he'd stuck his head in the pram, commented that she was pretty, and then he had virtually ignored her. He'd shown no interest in holding her. Lucy had put his behaviour down to him being a man. From what she'd seen, fathers rarely involved themselves with babies and left child-rearing to the mothers. That suited Lucy but, even so, she'd been disappointed that he hadn't been more forthcoming with his affections. Was this how he would be as a father to *their* children? Probably, she thought, but she supposed that was the way of the world.

'How was your mum today?' Winnie asked.

Lucy was irritated at the interruption of her thoughts and answered curtly, 'Fine, thanks.'

Her mind then drifted back to David. She'd told him about the engagement party that Winnie was throwing on Saturday afternoon. He'd gone quiet for a while afterwards. It must have hurt his feelings to be excluded from a big family celebration, especially when the *family* wasn't *real* family. Her heart went out to him and she deeply regretted mentioning it.

'Here, Lucy, how come you haven't got yourself a nice fella? A pretty girl like you, I would have thought you could have your pick.'

Lucy pursed her lips. Winnie was just making idle chat to pass the time but she didn't want to talk to her. She looked over the top of her book. 'I'm happy as I am,' she lied.

'Oh, right. Have you had your heart broken?'

'No.'

Rachel joined in. 'I don't blame you. Blokes are more trouble than they're worth. You're better off without them.'

'Yeah, maybe,' Winnie said, 'but most young women want to settle down and have a family.'

'I've got all the family I need right here,' Rachel said, gazing lovingly down at Martha.

'What about you, love?' Winnie asked. 'Don't you want a family?'

'No. I'm fine as I am,' Lucy lied again. But even the question tugged at her womb. She wanted a husband and children more than anything. Every waking moment of every day, she dreamed of being a mother and longed to hold a child in her arms. Today, for a couple of hours, pushing Martha around in her pram, she'd pretended the baby was hers and had felt so proud. But then when she'd handed Martha back to Rachel, reality had struck and she'd come crashing back down with a heavy bump. She had to have her own child soon before the yearnings drove her mad. And now all her hopes of having a husband and family were pinned on David.

10

On Thursday morning, Harry rushed around fulfilling his orders and collecting new stock. He had managed to squeeze what normally took him a whole day into just one morning. Now, at lunchtime, he sat at his kitchen table and spooned the last of the beef stew into his mouth. He looked over at Carmen. She'd hardly said a word and, though he was grateful for the peace and quiet, he knew that Cheryl visiting his mother was playing on Carmen's mind. They hadn't discussed it other than the few scribbled notes last night. But Harry warily broached the subject again. 'I don't suppose that Cheryl will go and see me mum until the weekend. Perhaps it would be better if we just told her the truth. It's better she hears it from us rather than me mum.'

Carmen shot him a look. 'Don't you dare say anything!' she said quickly. 'You promised me that you'd never tell the children, Harry, never. You'll have to stop Cheryl from seeing Edie and that'll be an end to it.'

'I don't know how to stop her. I've racked me brains thinking about it and I don't see how I can. That's why I think it's best that we tell Cheryl before me mum does.'

'No, Harry, I won't hear of it. You'll have to go and see your mother and tell her not to say anything to Cheryl.'

Harry coughed and spluttered on the mouthful of tea he'd just drunk. 'See my mother? I doubt she'd want to see me anymore than I want to see her,' he said, and he wiped his mouth with the back of his hand.

'It's not about what you want, is it?'

'No, but even if I did go and see her and ask her to keep quiet, why would she listen to me? If anything, that'll just make her even more determined to shoot her mouth off.'

'Well, I don't know, Harry, but she's your mother so you had better work out what you're going to do. I don't want to hear another word about it, is that clear?'

Go and see his mother. The thought left Harry with knots in his stomach. He hadn't seen her since the day he'd married Carmen and his mother had turned up to start trouble. She'd ruined the day and had reduced Carmen to tears, which was something rarely seen in his wife. That just went to show how upset Carmen had been! And if the truth be known, Harry had been deeply upset too, and embarrassed. He recalled the moment that his mother marched down the aisle of the church, wailing and crying that he shouldn't marry *that* woman. She'd even called Carmen a harlot! It had been the last straw when his mother had feigned a heart attack in order to halt the proceedings. Harry had seen straight through her fake illness. But the vicar had been duped by her act and so had some of the wedding guests. His mother had made Harry and Carmen appear cold and heartless. Yet, all the while, it was *she* who was the heartless one who'd set out to stop the wedding. And to top it all, the woman knew about Carmen being illegitimate. Harry was sure that his mother would readily expose it.

Somehow, he had to stop Cheryl from going to Balham. And he only had a day and a half to come up with a feasible plan.

Cheryl had looked over her shoulder at Ada at least a dozen times throughout the morning. Ada hadn't seemed to notice but Yvonne had.

'Has she been getting at you again?' her friend whispered.

'No, and even if she did, I'd soon put her back in her place. No, it's nothing like that. I'm thinking about how I'm going to approach her to ask about where my gran lives. You know what Ada is like. She's going to revel in me asking her for a favour.'

'I could ask for you?'

'It wouldn't make any difference, but thanks for offering. If I can get the address from her, I'm going to skive off this afternoon and go over there. You'll have to cover for me, tell Mr Mullen that I've gone home sick.'

'What if he asks what's wrong with you?'

'I dunno, Yvonne. Tell him it's me monthlies or something. That'll shut him up.'

Yvonne sniggered. 'Oh, I don't think I could say that!'

'Then say I've got a headache.'

'Do you think Ada will tell you what you want to know?'

'Oh, yeah, I'm sure she will. She'll love the idea of having something over me,' Cheryl answered. She looked over her shoulder again. Ada and her cronies were gossiping amongst themselves. Cheryl had the feeling they were talking about her. That was fine, she was used to women sniping about her behind her back. But she looked down her nose at their shiftiness. None of them, except Ada, would ever say anything to Cheryl's face. And if they did, they could expect a good mouthful of abuse back.

The minutes ticked by slowly for Cheryl. Eventually, it was lunchtime. As most of the women headed towards the canteen, Cheryl was quick to step in front of Ada. 'A word, please,' she said with an insincere smile and her head cocked to one side.

Ada's friends stood close by and watched as the woman leaned her face down towards Cheryl's. If Ada was trying to intimidate her, then it wasn't working. Cheryl feared no one, not even her mother.

'What?' Ada asked.

Cheryl turned to Ada's friends. 'Don't let me keep you from your lunch,' she told them.

Ada's friends sloped off, leaving her without an audience. 'What do you want?' she asked Cheryl, sounding impatient.

'I want to know Edie Hampton's address.'

A wicked grin spread across Ada's face. Just as Cheryl had expected, the woman was going to enjoy this and milk it for all it was worth.

'Oh, do ya now? So you've decided that you have got a gran in Balham after all. A gran who you and your lot have left for dead for all any of you care.'

'Are you going to give me the address or not?'

'Ask nicely.'

'Please.'

'I don't see why I should. Your gran is better off without you and yours and your stuck-up ways. My sister says that Edie is a kind woman, wouldn't hurt a fly and has a heart of gold. No wonder she don't have nothing to do with your family!'

'All right, Ada, you've said your piece. Now are you going to tell me where she lives?'

'Yeah, I'll tell you. But I'm warning you. If I hear from my sister that you've upset that nice old woman, I'll make sure your name is dirt in Battersea.'

Ada rattled off the address which Cheryl memorised easily. She dashed away without thanking Ada, clocked off and headed straight for the bus stop.

As she stood in the light, drizzling rain, she realised that she was beginning to feel nervous about introducing herself to Edie and she tried to imagine what sort of reception she would receive. Her gran might tell her to bugger off! But she might welcome her with open arms. Cheryl couldn't wait to meet her and she hoped her gran would be pleased to see her too.

Cheryl stood outside the neat, terraced house, her heart racing. The net curtains behind the windows looked pristine, as was the chalked doorstep and polished wooden door knocker. Edie Hampton was clearly a proud woman and capable of keeping her house in order, or at least the outside, if only for appearances sake.

She stepped towards the blue-painted door and realised that though it was chilly, her palm was clammy. She'd had plenty of time on the journey to Balham to consider how she would introduce herself to her gran, but as she knocked on the door, her mind went blank.

When no one answered, Cheryl was almost relieved. But

as she turned to walk away, the door opened and a short, white-haired old lady poked her head out.

'Can I help you?' she asked, her eyes squinting as she tried to focus on Cheryl.

Cheryl's mouth had gone very dry. 'Oh, erm – he-hello,' she stuttered. She found herself staring at the woman, amazed at the striking resemblance between her gran and her father.

'What do you want? You look too fancy to be begging for anything. Are you here on official business? Is it about me rent? I'm up to date.'

'Er, no, Mrs Hampton. I'm – erm – I'm Cheryl, Cheryl Hampton. Harry's daughter. Your granddaughter.' Cheryl gulped and waited with bated breath for the woman's response.

Edie pulled the door open wider and stepped towards Cheryl, her face screwed up quizzically as she studied Cheryl's features. 'My granddaughter, you say. Harry's daughter?'

'Yes, that's right. Sorry, I know this must be a shock for you.'

'You can say that again!'

Cheryl began to fish in her handbag. 'I can show you my National Identity Card, prove to you who I am?' she offered, holding the official document towards Edie.

'No need. I can see who you are. You're the spit of your mother. A lot shorter than Carmen, but you look just like her, especially with that black hair. You'd better come in.'

Cheryl followed her gran into the hallway and then through to the front room. She was pleasantly surprised to find a fire burning in the hearth, warming the room. She'd expected the house to smell of mothballs and to be dusty, but everything looked as shiny as a button, just like the exterior.

'There's fresh tea in the pot, sit yourself down,' her gran said, pointing to a cane chair by the fire.

Cheryl was glad of the heat on her legs. She pulled her gloves off and removed her hat, placing both on her lap. Edie had gone to the kitchen so Cheryl took advantage of being alone and surveyed the old woman's room. There were no photographs on display. And no pictures hung on the faded flowery wallpaper. A large ornately patterned, threadbare rug covered most of the floorboards and a dark wooden cased clock sat on the brick mantle between two heavy metal candlesticks. A big vase was on the oak sideboard and, next to that, Cheryl spotted a small, framed painting of a young man. She quietly placed her gloves and hat on the small table beside the chair and tiptoed over to the sideboard for a closer look.

'That's my Wilf, your grandfather,' Edie said.

Cheryl was startled at her gran's voice and spun round. 'I-I'm sorry, I wasn't prying,' she faltered, feeling flustered.

Edie held out a cup and saucer which rattled in her slightly trembling hand. ''Ere, a fresh cuppa.'

Cheryl took the cup and sat back in the armchair. 'Is my grandad—?'

'Dead,' Edie interrupted. 'He died when I was carrying your father. Pneumonia, they said.'

'Oh, I'm sorry.'

'How is he, your father?'

'He's very well.'

Edie sniffed. 'Does he know you're here?'

Cheryl shrugged. 'I think he knows that I was planning on visiting you.'

'And he allowed you to come?'

'No, not exactly.'

'So, what brings you here? Looking at the way you're dolled up, I shouldn't think you've come for money.'

Cheryl cast her eyes downwards, embarrassed at being overdressed as usual. 'No, I'm not here for money,' she said quietly.

'What you 'ere for, then? I mean, none of you have bothered with me for years, so why now?'

'I didn't know about you. I only found out the other day.'

'What do you mean, *you didn't know about me*? Oh, don't tell me – your mother and father told you that I was dead. I'm right, ain't I?'

Cheryl felt awful but she nodded her head.

Her gran's thin lips set in a straight line. 'That doesn't surprise me.'

'Why would they have lied to me my whole life?'

Edie rolled her eyes in just the same way that Cheryl had seen her father do many times. 'They ain't told you, have they?' her gran asked.

'Told me what?'

'Well, well, well. I'm amazed that they've managed to keep you in the dark all these years.'

'Please, tell me, in the dark about what?'

'You should ask them, but I'm warning you, it's not nice.'

'They won't tell me anything and, anyway, why should I believe a word they say? They lied to me about you being, you know, dead,' Cheryl said, feeling uncomfortable at using that fatal word.

'Does Errol know about me?'

'No. I haven't seen him but I'm sure that when I tell him,

he'll want to meet you. You know about Errol, then. But did you know that you had a granddaughter?'

'Yes, dear, I heard about you being born. It broke my heart that I couldn't see you.'

'Please, Gran, tell me what happened.'

Edie placed her cup and saucer on the table and slowly pushed herself out of the armchair opposite Cheryl. Though the woman wasn't as frail or feeble as Cheryl had expected, she could see her gran was stiff with arthritis.

Edie went to the sideboard, opened a door and pulled out a biscuit tin. She came back and sat down with the tin on her lap. She looked at Cheryl with pale-blue rheumy eyes and asked, 'Are you sure you want to know? It's ugly.'

Cheryl nodded her head emphatically.

'All right, but you're not going to thank me for what I'm going to say.'

'I just want the truth, warts an' all,' Cheryl said eagerly. She shifted forward to sit on the edge of the seat, waiting in anticipation of what her gran was about to impart.

Edie sat back and gazed towards the window, saying firmly, 'I won't mince my words. Your mother is a slut.'

Cheryl's mouth opened in shock but no words came out.

'And your mother's mother was a slut too. It must run in the family. I hope you take after my side and not theirs.' Edie turned from the window and looked back at Cheryl. 'Don't sit there with your mouth gaping, you ain't heard the worst of it yet. I suppose you think you've got Spanish blood. I should imagine that's what you've been told?'

'Erm, yes, from my mum's side.'

'Your mother has about as much Spanish blood in her as a flippin' goldfish! She ain't told you the truth cos she's ashamed and so she bleedin' well should be! Your mother, who acts like she's so high and mighty, was born out of wedlock. Her mother had a one-night stand with a gypsy and that's how Carmen came to be. What do you think of that, eh?'

Cheryl was speechless. She didn't know what to think and stared blankly at her gran.

'You would have thought that Carmen would have tried to do better than her mother but she followed in her footsteps. Errol, your brother, was born just four months after your mum and dad got married. What does that tell you?'

'I can't believe it,' Cheryl mumbled. 'But at least they were married.'

'Oh, there's more. I ain't even got to the best bit yet.' Edie opened the biscuit tin on her lap. 'The rest of the story is in here,' she said as she handed the tin to Cheryl. 'I had two boys. My Wilf was born first and named after his father. Harry came along three years later. They were both smart boys, Wilf more so than your father. They were good an' all but they were always scrapping with each other – like brothers do, I suppose. Your father always wanted what your brother had. Wilf was a gentler boy than Harry and shy too. Harry, he always had the gift of the gab and could charm the birds down from the trees. I don't suppose he's changed,' Edie said with a small chuckle. Her expression then quickly changed and she looked stern again. 'I suppose his charm is what attracted your mother. But she was Wilf's girl. Wilf and Carmen were engaged and planned to get married. I was against it. I never liked your mother and didn't think that she was good enough for my Wilf. But he loved her. Anyway, the Great War happened and Wilf was quick to volunteer to join up. He went off to basic training and the next time we saw him was on a route march through Regent's Park. He looked so handsome.' Edie smiled warmly as she retold the memory and her eyes went back to gazing towards the window. But then they snapped round to Cheryl again. 'Your mother didn't come to the park with me to see Wilf,' Edie said bitterly. 'Unknown to me or anyone else, she was conniving to marry your father.'

'But I thought she was engaged to Wilf.'

'She was! And as it turned out, she was also in the family way. When I found out what was going on, I wrote to Wilf and told him. He sent a letter back, begging me to stop the wedding. It's in there, in that tin, all of it. You can see for yourself.'

Cheryl thumbed through the postcards and letters written on yellowed paper. The writing was difficult to discern but she read one letter from Wilf that said the child in Carmen's stomach was his. Harry had stolen his wife and child! 'This letter, Gran,' Cheryl said, holding it out. 'The child. Is that Errol?'

'Yes, dear. Wilf thought that the baby was his. Harry denied it. But, like I said, your mother is a slut. She was cavorting with both my boys at the same time. Either one of them could have fathered Errol. We'll never really know the truth.'

'Blimey, this is shocking!'

'I tried to stop the wedding. I got myself so upset that I had a funny turn in the church. Your mother and father didn't care. In fact, your mother turned on the waterworks and I was shown the door. The next day, Carmen showed up on my doorstep and told me I'd never see Harry again and that I was dead to them both.'

'And that was it?'

'Yeah, I suppose it was. I tried again to see them. Once I'd heard that Errol had been born, I went round to the house but your father slammed the door in my face. And then when Wilf was killed, I went to see Harry, but Carmen wouldn't let me over the doorstep and Harry told me to bugger off.'

'Wilf was killed?'

'Yes, in France.' Edie's eyes filled with tears. She drew in a sharp breath and said, 'I was told that he died a hero. He put himself in front of another soldier to save the man's life. But he didn't die a hero. He died a broken man. You can read between the lines in his letters. He didn't want to live. He didn't feel he had anything worth living for. I know my boy. He deliberately put himself in front of that soldier purely because he *wanted* to die. And that's because of what Harry and your mother did to him.' Edie pulled a handkerchief from the sleeve of her cardigan and wiped her nose. 'Now you understand why your mother and father didn't want you seeing me. I've nothing to hide. It's them who ought to be ashamed of themselves.'

Cheryl was crying now too. It had been a lot to take in but the truth was clear to see in Wilf's letters. She wasn't surprised at how callous her mother had been but she'd never have expected her dad to have behaved so despicably. 'I'm so sorry, Gran,' she muttered through her tears.

'It's not your fault, you ain't got nothing to be sorry for. Get yourself a hankie, there's a clean one in the sideboard drawer.'

Cheryl went to the sideboard and tried to gather her thoughts. She blew her nose and came back to sit down. After carefully placing the letters in the tin, she handed it back to her gran. 'My mum and dad left you with no one and all because they wanted to hide what they'd done. Gran, that's awful.'

'Your mother was behind it. Harry would never have turned his back on me if it weren't for her making him do it,' Edie said, her lip curling in disgust. 'But don't you worry about me. I've looked after myself all this time, I'm more than capable.'

'I can see that but it's not the point! You've done nothing wrong. You didn't deserve to be ignored by the family and they've deprived me of having a gran.'

Edie's face softened. 'Well, you've got one now. And in my books, a gran should bake and stuff her grandkids with cake. Have a look in my larder. There's a nice bit of sponge cake. Well, I say nice. It's as nice as I can make it with these stupid rations. Go and get us both a slice and we'll have a fresh cuppa too.'

Cheryl did as her gran instructed and then returned to the cosy front room with the cake and tea. She sat down but, before eating, she asked, 'Gran, when I was in the kitchen, I noticed you don't have a shelter out the back. Do you go to a public shelter? I hear a lot of people are using the underground train platforms, even though they're not supposed to. Is that where you go?'

Her gran chuckled again. 'I stay in me bed nice and warm. Best place to be.'

'But that's not safe!'

'If him upstairs calls you in, there's nothing we can do about it. I've had a good innings and if the Hun is going to drop a bomb on me, then I want to make sure I die in me own bed and not stuffed in somewhere with a load of strangers.'

'I can organise you a shelter for the backyard if you like?'

'No, thanks. Like I said, I'm happy in me bed. If I die there, at least my Wilf will know where to find me.'

Cheryl bit into the dry sponge slice. She'd been horrified to hear her mother being called a slut but now she understood why. She'd been unsure of her gran at first but she'd quickly warmed to her. The poor woman, she thought. Edie had lost both her boys and her husband. Though she seemed too proud to admit it, Cheryl thought her gran must be lonely. But she wouldn't be anymore. Cheryl would make sure of it. As she struggled to swallow the cake, she thought how cruel her parents had been and a knot of anger formed in her stomach. Their secret was out now and Cheryl wasn't sure that she'd ever be able to forgive them.

'Where on earth could she have got to?' Carmen asked Harry as she paced the kitchen floor. 'It's not like her not to come straight home from work. Are you sure she wasn't in the pub?'

'I'm sure. None of the girls were there this evening. Maybe they've gone to another pub.'

'No, I doubt it. Something's not right, Harry.'

They heard the front door open and Carmen rushed from the room and into the passageway. Harry heard his wife's disappointed voice when she said, 'Oh, it's you. Have you seen your sister?'

'No, not for a few days. Is she all right?'

'I don't know. She's not come home from work.'

'Is that all? She'll be home soon. Is there any tea in the pot?'

'Yes. Your father's in the front room. Go and sit down, I'll fetch you a cuppa.'

Errol strolled into the room, his imposing frame seeming to fill it. 'Wotcha, Dad. Mum's a bit worked up.'

'I know, Son. I think all this bombing has got her worried. And it doesn't help that you don't bother showing your face from one day to the next. Spare a thought for your mother, will you. Stick your head through the front door a bit more often.'

Harry saw his son inhale deeply.

'You're inconsiderate. You know how much your mother worries.'

'And here we go again,' Errol said as the sirens wailed into action.

Carmen darted into the front room. 'Where is she? She should be home.'

'I'm sure she's with her friends and they will be making their way to the nearest shelter, just like we're about to do. Come on,' Harry said, ushering his wife towards the back door in the kitchen.

'No, Harry. I'm not going in there. I'll wait for Cheryl.'

'Don't be daft. Cheryl's a sensible girl. She'll be looking after herself.'

'Dad's right, Mum. I'll go out and have a look for her. You go with Dad,' Errol offered.

'You'll do no such thing! I'm not having both my kids on the missing list. You'll get in the shelter with me and your father.'

'I'll be fine.' Errol said, heading to the front door, ignoring Carmen's pleas for him to come back.

Harry pulled his wife towards the kitchen and they trudged through the small back garden to the Anderson shelter. A puddle had formed in the middle of the floor and the place wreaked of damp soil. But the dreary state of the shelter was the least of his worries. Harry wouldn't let on to his wife but he was secretly worried about Cheryl too. He'd seen Yvonne, Carol and Anne in the Battersea Tavern. When he'd asked after Cheryl, Yvonne had appeared twitchy. She'd mumbled something about Cheryl going shopping for a new dress for the party on Saturday. It didn't ring true to Harry. He'd already heard his daughter waxing lyrical about the red dress she was going to wear. He had a sneaking suspicion that Cheryl had gone to see his mother. If that was the case, the air raids and long nights in the shelter were going to seem like a walk in the park compared to what was about to be unleashed on his family.

11

On Friday morning, Winnie pulled a tray of freshly baked sausage rolls from the oven. Her stomach grumbled at the delicious aroma. As she transferred them to a wire rack to cool, she resisted the temptation to eat one.

'Something smells nice,' Rachel said as she came into the kitchen carrying Martha in her arms.

'Sausage rolls for the party tomorrow, thanks to Harry giving me the meat. I've made some Scotch eggs too.'

'Blimey, your customers are in for a treat.'

'Indeed. You know how hard sausages and eggs are to come by. He's a good man,' Winnie said. She could feel her cheeks flush at the mention of Harry and she turned away from Rachel, hoping that the girl hadn't noticed.

'It's a shame that Errol doesn't take after his father,' Rachel moaned.

'It is, but at least Errol behaves himself in my pub.' Winnie recalled Harry mentioning his doubts about being Errol's father. If that was the case, then it went a long way to explaining why the two men were so different. ''Ere, let me take Martha and you can put the kettle on.'

Winnie sat down with the baby and gazed down into her little face. She searched Martha's features and saw a resemblance to David. The thought of David made her stomach churn. He hadn't been back but Winnie had a feeling that he would be. She'd heard from her customers that there'd been several sightings of him around Battersea so she knew that she'd see him again. Her heart ached and she missed him dreadfully. But she'd never forgive him for what he'd done to Rachel and reminded herself that he was just like his father, a horrid man.

Lucy came into the kitchen, dressed and looking ready to face the day, unlike Winnie, still in her nightie and dressing gown, and Rachel, who was wearing the same creased clothes she'd worn yesterday and throughout the night in the cellar.

'Morning,' Lucy greeted them cheerfully.

'Morning, love. I don't know where you find your energy. Look at the state of me and Rachel. We're knackered after last night's raid.'

'Me an' all but a girl's got to keep up her appearances.'

'Oh yeah, who for?' Winnie asked with a chuckle. 'Out to impress someone, are you?'

'No, not at all. But I've got my standards.'

'I hope you're not implying that me and Winnie don't?' Rachel spluttered sharply.

'No, of course I'm not. You're busy with a baby and Winnie is – erm—'

'Is what?' Winnie cut in.

'Erm – older,' Lucy answered, sounding uncomfortable.

Well, Winnie couldn't argue with that. And being *older* was all the more reason for her to feel so silly about having a crush on Harry. Surely that's all it was, just a silly crush?

'You're brave saying that about Winnie,' Rachel whispered.

'No, she's right, love. I am getting on compared to you two. But that doesn't mean that us oldies don't like to look nice too. So on that note, I'm going to get dressed. And Lucy, you can watch Martha while Rachel has a wash and changes her clothes.'

'But, I'm going out. I could take Martha with me, if you like?'

'Where are you off to at this time of the morning?' Winnie asked.

'Just to check on me mum and then I thought I'd clear the cobwebs and go for a walk.'

Winnie's eyes narrowed as she looked at Lucy. The girl was acting cagey. And now that Winnie came to think of it, Lucy seemed to be visiting her mother a lot, which seemed odd, especially as Lucy had said that she didn't get on with her stepdad. 'Perhaps Rachel could go with you? It's been ages since she's been outside the front door.'

'Oh, I don't know about that, Win. What if I were to bump into David?' Rachel protested.

'That's highly unlikely. You know he's never been an early riser,' Winnie answered. She looked over at Lucy and noticed that the colour had drained from her face. She was convinced that the girl was hiding something. 'It'd be nice for you to have a bit of company on your walk, wouldn't it?'

'Yes, but I could be at my mum's for a while and she won't thank me for calling in unannounced with visitors.'

'I thought you was only going to check on her?' Winnie pushed.

'Yeah, I am, but I'll have to stay and have a cuppa. She'd get upset if I didn't.'

'Rachel won't mind waiting while you have a quick cuppa with your mum. Hilda lives on the next street. Rachel could pop in and see Hilda and then you can both go off on your walk. It'll do Rachel the world of good and I'd much rather she was out with you than out by herself.'

Rachel's face brightened. 'Actually, that's not a bad idea,' she said. 'I haven't seen much of Hilda lately, not since she got involved with her voluntary work. I'm sure Martha would like to say a quick hello to her gran. And I really could do with a change of scene.'

Winnie looked at Lucy to gauge her reaction and though the girl smiled, Winnie could see that it didn't reach her eyes. But she couldn't think of any reason why Lucy wouldn't want Rachel to accompany her – unless Lucy was lying about what she was really planning to do this morning.

Cheryl hooked her arm through Yvonne's as they headed towards the factory. 'Thanks for letting me stay the night at yours,' she told her friend.

'That's all right. You know you're always welcome, as long as you don't mind sharing my bed. Or being under it like we was last night.'

'It was a bit of a squeeze but I wouldn't have got any decent kip in our Anderson at home. I'm just grateful that I didn't have to face my mum and dad.'

'Are you going home this evening or do you want my brother to drop another note at your house?' Yvonne asked.

'I suppose I should go home. I can't avoid them forever but I'm still furious at them both. And wait till Errol finds out. He'll do his nut.'

'Do you think you should tell him? It could upset him to hear that your dad might not be his dad.'

'He's got a right to know. I couldn't keep something like this from him. That would make me as bad as my mum and dad,' Cheryl answered.

A brisk wind blew around the corner of the street causing Cheryl's coat to billow open. She pulled it back around her and buttoned the front. When she looked back up, she saw Ada outside the factory gates. 'Great, this is all I need,' Cheryl mumbled.

'Try and take no notice of anything she says,' Yvonne advised.

'Don't worry, I'm in the mood for a fight and if Ada wants one, she's going to bloody well get one. Come on,' Cheryl said. She looped her arm back through Yvonne's and picked up her pace, almost dragging Yvonne along the street with her.

As they neared the gates, Cheryl braced herself for Ada's scathing remarks but she noticed that the woman's eyes were puffy and she was pulling hard on a cigarette. Instead of her usual confrontational manner, Ada cast her eyes downward and turned away from Cheryl.

'Something's up with her,' Cheryl whispered to Yvonne.

'Probably got a good hiding off her old man again last night.'

'No, it's not that. Ada has had thick lips and black eyes before off her old man but it's never shut her up.'

'Well, whatever it is, it's not your problem,' Yvonne said.

'Hmm, maybe not. You go in and clock on. I'm going to have a quick word with her.'

'She won't thank you for it.'

Cheryl shrugged and turned on her heel to head back outside the gates. She found Ada lighting another cigarette and asked, 'Aren't you coming in? It's a bit nippy out here.'

Ada didn't answer and turned her back to Cheryl.

Undeterred, Cheryl walked round to face Ada. 'Thanks for telling me about my gran.'

Ada blew smoke in the air. Sounding nonchalant, she said, 'Better late than never.'

Now Cheryl knew that something was very wrong with Ada. She had given the woman the perfect opportunity to say something derisive but Ada hadn't taken the bait. 'Are you all right?' she asked.

'What's it got to do with you?'

'Nothing. But you don't seem yourself.'

'I'm not.'

'Can I help?' Cheryl offered.

'I doubt it. Not unless you can tell me where Arthur is. My boy's been reported missing in action,' Ada answered, her voice cracking.

Cheryl normally had no time for the woman but her heart went out to her. She'd sensed straightaway that something wasn't right with Ada but she hadn't expected to hear such upsetting news about Arthur. She knew him, not well, but enough to say hello to. Arthur had been in Errol's year at school, a nice lad by all accounts. 'I'm so sorry, Ada. I don't know what to say.'

'There's nothing you can say. I've just got to get on with it and try not to think the worst.'

'Do you want to go home? I can explain to Mr Mullen.'

'No, I'll be in, in a tick. I need to keep busy. There's no point me sitting at home and worrying,' Ada said firmly.

She threw her cigarette to the ground and stubbed it out with the flat heel of her worn shoe, then immediately lit another. 'I'm running short of fags, huh; all I need at a time like this.'

'Don't worry about that. I'll get you some from me dad.'

Ada looked down at Cheryl. 'Why would you do anything nice for me? I don't need your sympathy or any charity from your family.'

'I know, but in times like this, we've got to pull together.'

Much to Cheryl's surprise, Ada burst into tears. Cheryl didn't have a handkerchief on her and wasn't sure how to react to Ada's sobs. 'Shall I go and fetch someone for you?' she offered, thinking of the woman's old cronies in the factory.

'No, I'm fine,' Ada said and sniffed. 'Sorry for snapping at you.'

Cheryl shrugged and offered a small smile. 'Come on, let's clock on before we're late,' she said.

Ada nodded and the women walked into the factory together. After years of bickering, it seemed that Cheryl and Ada had finally made an unspoken truce. But Cheryl knew that her peace wouldn't last long, for she had a very different battle to face tonight. One with her deceitful mother and father.

Lucy walked along the street with Rachel by her side. Rachel was nervously chatting but Lucy didn't hear a single word. She was too busy looking for any sight of David, though she knew it was unlikely that she'd see him near the Latchmere baths, as they'd arranged to meet in Battersea Park. She worried that when she didn't show up, David would think she'd stood him up and wouldn't be happy. But she had no way of getting word to him.

She glanced into the pram at Martha. The baby was sleeping soundly and looked so angelic. Lucy wished that she was pushing the pram and that Martha was her child. She thought she'd make a better mother than Rachel and the child would grow up with a father. Instead, poor Martha would never really know David. It wasn't fair on David either but at least, one day, he'd have the opportunity to be a proper father to their children.

'Well, what do you think?' Rachel's voice broke into Lucy's thoughts.

'Erm – sorry, what did you say?' she asked.

'I said, do you think that Jan and Terry will expect an engagement present?'

'Oh – erm – no, I shouldn't think so,' Lucy answered. She hadn't even thought of buying them something. She had never met Jan and she hardly knew Terry.

'I feel awful not getting them anything but I've not been out,' Rachel said.

Her words floated over Lucy's head. She saw a figure turn the corner. For a fleeting moment, she thought it was David and her heart skipped a beat. But she'd been mistaken. They were near her mother's house now and Lucy considered running all the way to the park and back again. But she knew there wasn't time to cover the distance. If only she could let David know that she hadn't deliberately let him down!

Lucy, feeling annoyed with herself, looked round at Rachel who was jabbering on about something. *This is silly* she thought. If she was to become David's wife, then she needed to put him first!

'I've got to go,' she blurted impulsively. Lucy quickly spun and darted off towards the park.

She heard Rachel call, 'Hang on. Where are you going?'

Lucy ignored her and carried on. She'd think of a lame excuse later, one that would cover her actions. But for now, she only wanted to be with David.

Twenty minutes later, she scanned the boating lake area, sorely disappointed when there was no sign of David. She hadn't been very late and had expected to find him waiting for her. But the weather had taken a turn for the worse so she didn't think badly of him for not hanging around. Feeling deflated, and in the pouring rain, she headed back to the pub. Her mind was completely occupied with where David could be and how she could contact him. Stupidly, she'd never asked him exactly where he was staying. She could kick herself. And to top it all, now she had to find an excuse to explain away her sudden running away from Rachel.

By the time Lucy reached the back door of the Battersea Tavern, she was soaked through and cold. She shivered as she put her key in the lock and quietly slipped inside. Her wet hair dripped down her back as she tiptoed up the stairs, hoping to avoid Winnie and Rachel. When she reached the upstairs landing, she could hear their voices drifting out from the kitchen.

'I don't know, Win, she was acting strange all morning. Like she was distracted or something,' Rachel said.

'I've got a feeling she's up to something. Gawd knows what but I'm sure it involves a bloke.'

'Why would she want to hide it from us?'

'I don't know, love. Unless she's seeing someone she shouldn't be,' Winnie replied.

'What, you mean a married man?'

'Could be. But I won't have any of those sorts of shenanigans going on under my roof. I run a respectable establishment and that's how I'm going to keep it.'

Lucy, wide-eyed, padded to her room. So, they thought she was seeing a married man! Neither of the witches seemed to suspect that it was David. Quickly she stripped off her sodden clothes and hung them over the back of the chair. She put her coat on a hanger. It was so wet, it would take days to dry properly. After throwing on her dressing gown and rubbing her hair with a towel, Lucy sat on the edge of her bed and tensed when she heard a knock on the door.

'Come in,' she called.

Winnie opened the door and eyed her dubiously. 'What happened to you? You left Rachel all alone. Thank goodness Hilda was able to walk her home.'

'Yes, I'm sorry about that. I don't know what came over me.'

'What do you mean?'

'It was horrible, Winnie. I thought I saw my stepdad coming out of the house. I panicked and ran off. I wasn't thinking clearly, sorry. Is Rachel all right?'

'Yeah, she's fine. Are you?'

'I am now. I feel terrible about running off like that. I'm a grown woman; I shouldn't be scared of him but...' Lucy lied, forcing tears out of her eyes.

'It's all right, love. Don't worry and don't upset yourself. No harm done, eh.'

'Thanks, Winnie. Can you tell Rachel I'm sorry?'

'Of course. You get yourself warmed up and dressed. We're opening in half an hour.'

Winnie gently closed the door behind her and Lucy sighed with relief. She walked towards the window and looked at the dark and cloudy sky. Hopefully, throughout the morning, the rain would ease. Because Lucy had a plan for when the pub closed after lunch. Even if it meant that she had to visit every bed and breakfast in Battersea, she intended to find her fella.

12

At lunchtime, Yvonne asked Cheryl, 'Are you coming to the canteen?'

'No, I want to find my brother,' Cheryl whispered in reply.

'I'll come with you.'

Cheryl had guessed that Yvonne would. Her friend would never miss an opportunity of seeing Errol.

Outside, the rain had abated but dirty water that had pooled on the ground splashed the back of Cheryl's stockings. 'I suppose the cloud cover will make it difficult for the Luftwaffe to attack tonight. You never know, we might get a decent night's sleep for a change.'

'I wouldn't count on it. It looks like it's brightening up,' Yvonne said, pointing to the sky behind them. 'Where are we going to start looking for Errol?' she asked.

'I've got a feeling he might be in the pub near that doll's shop that you like.'

'Oh, blimey, Cheryl, I'm not sure about going in there! I've heard it's pretty rough.'

'Don't worry. I'll pop my head in and look for him. You don't have to come in,' Cheryl reassured her. She wasn't keen on going in there either but she reckoned that no one would dare say or do anything to the sister of Errol Hampton.

Once they reached the pub, Yvonne looked anxious.

'It's all right, Yvonne. I won't be more than two minutes. If Errol is in there, I'll get him to come out,' Cheryl said.

With trepidation, but holding her head high, Cheryl pulled the door open. She was immediately hit by the smell of tobacco smoke wafting out and the low murmur of men's voices. Stepping inside, she squinted her eyes against the dim lights. The pub was nothing like the cheery atmosphere that she always found in the Battersea Tavern. It was exactly how Errol had told her it would be – spit and sawdust.

As the door closed behind her, the pub fell deathly quiet and all eyes stared at her. Cheryl looked along the bar for any sign of her brother. Nothing. She turned her head to look from corner to corner but there was no sign of him. Just as she was about to leave, a bloke called to her.

'Are you touting for business, darling?'

'No, I'm not!' she answered incredulously.

A small ripple of laughter went around the pub. Cheryl could feel her cheeks burning. She wished her brother were here!

'If you're looking for someone, Frankie over there could do with a good woman.'

The laughter became louder now. Cheryl looked towards where the man was pointing and saw Frankie – a one-legged, toothless old man who blew her a kiss while gazing at her leeringly.

Cheryl's stomach turned but she announced, 'I'm looking for my brother, Errol Hampton.'

The laughter stopped instantly and most of the men averted

their eyes and carried on with supping their ales. The landlord cleared his throat before speaking. 'He'll be here any minute. Would you like to wait out the back for him, miss?'

'No, thank you,' Cheryl answered and spun on her heel. She couldn't get out of the pub quickly enough.

Pleased to be back outside in the fresh air, she was relieved to find Errol talking to a crimson-faced Yvonne. 'Ah, there you are,' she said as she walked towards them.

'Did you get any stick in there?' Errol asked.

'No, not really.'

'Yvonne said you need to talk to me about something. Do you want to come in for a drink?'

'No, not in there. But can we go to the Corner Café?' Cheryl asked.

'If you want,' Errol replied, shrugging.

The café was just a few doors down from the pub. As Errol walked in, Yvonne tugged on the arm of Cheryl's coat and asked, 'Shall I wait out here for you?'

'No, don't be daft. Come in.'

Cheryl and Yvonne sat opposite Errol. He lit a cigarette and offered one to Yvonne, who quickly shook her head.

'Give us a couple of packets of those,' Cheryl said, pointing at the cigarettes.

'You don't smoke,' Errol replied.

'I know, but Ada at work, her Arthur is missing in action. I know it ain't much but a couple of packets of fags is better than nothing.'

Errol didn't argue. He pulled three packets from his inside coat pocket and threw them onto the table, saying, 'That's a shame about Arthur. I've always had a lot of time for the bloke. Here, take these for his mum. That's all I've got. Now, what's this all about? You ain't dragged me away from the pub to ask me for smokes.'

Before Cheryl could explain, the waitress appeared to take their order. Errol asked for three cups of tea, a large plate of chips and two sticky buns. 'That all right for you both?' he asked Cheryl.

'Yes, thanks, smashing.'

The waitress went off to the kitchen and Cheryl leaned forward across the table towards her brother. She'd been desperate to tell him about their gran but now she felt butterflies in her stomach and her jaw clenched.

'What's the matter, Sis?' he asked, clearly sensing her discomfort.

'I've got something to tell you but I'm not sure how you're going to take it.'

'You'd better not be up the duff,' Errol hissed, his eyes glaring angrily. 'Cos I'll kill whoever did it to you.'

'No, of course I'm not! And if I was, you'd be the last person I'd tell. It's about our gran.'

Errol stubbed out his cigarette. 'What gran?' he asked.

'Our gran, Edie Hampton, who is alive and well and living in Balham.'

'Eh? I thought she died donkey's years ago.'

'Yeah, that's what Mum and Dad would have us believe but they've lied to us. I've met her, Errol; it's true.'

'I don't understand. Why would they have lied to us?'

Cheryl drew in a long breath, suddenly unsure of how her brother would react and worried that he'd take the news badly. 'They didn't want us finding out their secrets. So they lied to keep us from our gran.'

'What secrets?'

'That mum was illegitimate. Her dad was a gypsy who her mum had a brief fling with.'

'Eh? Is that all? That's no big deal.'

'No, that's not all,' Cheryl answered and swallowed hard. 'Our dad, he had a brother, Wilf. Our mum and Wilf were engaged to be married but then Wilf signed up with the army during the Great War. Then Mum married our dad instead and Wilf got killed.'

There was a long, silent pause, and Cheryl added, 'Wilf might be your dad.'

Errol's eyes widened and, for a moment, Cheryl feared he was about to lose his violent temper. But then a smile spread across his face and he started to chuckle. 'So, Harry Hampton ain't my dad, he's my spineless little uncle.'

'I don't know, Errol. He could be your dad – or Wilf could be.'

'I've always known it; I swear I have. I knew there was something not right. Now it makes sense. He ain't me dad, Wilf is.'

'You don't know that for sure.'

'Yeah, I do. And I'll tell you what, it's the best news I've had in ages.'

The waitress appeared again and placed their cups of tea in front of them. Then she quickly returned with the chips and buns. Cheryl told Yvonne to get stuck in.

'Why is it good news?' Cheryl asked.

'Cos I only show him any respect because he's my dad. Now he can go and take a running jump. Let's face it, he's never been bothered about me. You've always been his favourite. Do Mum and Dad know that we know?'

'Not yet. I've been too upset to face them. But I'm going to have it out with them later. Will you be there with me?'

'Yeah, I'll be there tonight, for you, but that's it. I'm packing me stuff and going.'

Cheryl was quick to respond. 'No, please, Errol, don't leave,' she pleaded and reached across the table for her brother's hand.

He gripped it reassuringly. 'Don't worry, I'll always be here for you. It's just them I can't stomach. *Uncle* Harry and Mum have spent their whole lives screaming and shouting at each other. I'll be glad to see the back of it.'

'But he *could* be your dad and even if he isn't, he's still your uncle, still family.'

'I don't care, Sis. The bloody pair of 'em are as bad as each other.'

Cheryl had to agree with her brother. She'd spent so much of her life in her bedroom hiding away from her parents' arguments. It hadn't been a joyous or harmonious upbringing. Though when she'd dared to moan about it, her mother had rammed it down her throat that Cheryl was luckier than most as she hadn't wanted for anything. But Cheryl had wanted for something. She had wanted the love and affection that her mother withheld. And though she was spoilt rotten by her father, she'd always sensed the resentment that it had caused in her mother. Perhaps Errol had the right idea. Maybe she should pack her bags and leave her mum and dad to get on with it. 'Where will you go?' she asked him.

'I've got a small flat off Westbridge Road. Nice place. I'll take you round there soon, so you know where I am.'

'You've got a place already? Why didn't you say?'

'I didn't want to upset Mum. Where do you think I am most nights?'

'I don't know, on mates' sofas, I assumed.' Cheryl sipped

her tea and looked over the top of her cup at Errol. 'Can I move in with you?' she asked in her sweetest voice.

'No.'

'Oh, go on. I'd keep the place clean and do all your cooking for you.'

'I don't need a housekeeper.'

'Please, Errol. I'd be no trouble. You wouldn't even know I was there.'

'I said no. Anyway, there's not enough room. Steph lives with me.'

Cheryl huffed. 'Stephanie Reynolds, huh, so you'll have a tart living with you but not your own sister,' she said sulkily, her lips pouting.

'Oi, Steph ain't a tart so button it.'

Cheryl could tell by her brother's tone of voice that she'd pushed her luck with her last comment. 'Sorry. Can I just stay with you until I find my own place?'

'No, and that's an end to it. Pass me a chip.'

Yvonne pushed the plate over towards Errol. Her cheeks were flaming red when she asked, 'Are you going to the party in the Battersea Tavern tomorrow?'

'Yeah, I said I'd keep an eye on this one,' he answered, nodding towards Cheryl.

'Are you bringing Stephanie?' Cheryl asked.

'Of course.'

Cheryl glanced sideways at Yvonne and could see the disappointment on her face.

'Right, ladies, enjoy your lunch. I'm off,' Errol said as he scraped back his chair. He left some money on the table and sauntered out.

'See you at home later,' Cheryl called after him as a

reminder. She'd been pleasantly surprised at how well he'd taken the news though he hadn't asked after their gran. She hadn't realised he'd held so much resentment towards their dad but, thinking back, she could see it now. Their father had always been harder on Errol and it was always him who would get the blame for their naughtiness. She'd assumed it was because he was the eldest but now she saw it differently. In fact, there'd been a wedge between her dad and Errol for years, a distance she couldn't put her finger on. And the more she thought about it, the more it made her wonder if her father knew that he wasn't Errol's real dad.

Harry looked across the kitchen table at his wife. She glared back at him but remained silent. No supper was simmering on the stove. No kettle boiling. Just a thick tension hung in the air as they waited for Cheryl to come home.

The previous night, once the planes and bombs had quietened, Harry had slipped back into the house and found a note from Yvonne's brother, shoved through the door, explaining that Cheryl was staying the night at their house. Harry had known instantly that his daughter had been to see her gran and was too upset to come home. And since he'd told Carmen about it, his wife hadn't spoken a word.

Harry drew in a long breath and got up from the table and walked through to the front room. He glanced through the net curtains and tensed when he saw Cheryl. She was leaning against a garden wall a few houses down. He wondered what she was doing but it soon became clear when he saw Errol walking towards her. She'd been waiting for her brother and now Harry thought that the situation had gone from bad to worse. His heart began to hammer. He couldn't help feeling nervous of his son's temperament, especially now that Errol was a good few inches taller than him – and broader too. If his son's explosive temper got out of control, there was little or nothing that Harry could do to calm him. And he knew from experience that Errol had no qualms about facing up to him. They'd locked horns on many occasions, Errol only backing down when Carmen had intervened.

Harry walked back through to the kitchen; his fists clenched. 'They're here,' he said solemnly to Carmen.

Again, his wife met him with silence.

He heard the front door open and tried to appear calm to hide his anxiety. Cheryl marched in first, looking splendid but fierce. Errol ambled in behind her. He didn't meet Harry's eyes as he strolled across the kitchen and then leaned against the sink before lighting up a cigarette. Harry was sure this would antagonise Carmen. She hated the smell of tobacco burning and had often thrown Errol out into the yard to smoke. But still his wife sat, tight-lipped.

Cheryl broke the strained stillness. 'You've probably worked out that I've been to see my gran, who enlightened me about your lies and deceit,' she said coldly.

Harry pulled out the seat opposite his wife and sat down. He held his hands on his lap to hide the fact that they were trembling. This was ridiculous, he thought, afraid of his own kids. Scared of Errol kicking off. Worried about Carmen being upset with him. He cleared his throat, then said firmly, 'Whatever me and your mother did in the past, we did for good reason and we don't have to answer to you. So be careful what you say, young lady, and show me and your mother the respect we deserve.'

'*Respect?*' Cheryl spat. 'You lost my respect the moment

I discovered I have a gran who you abandoned just so that you could keep your horrible secrets to yourselves. And what about me and Errol? Don't our feelings count? Don't you think we would have liked to know our gran? You're selfish, the pair of you, and I'm so ashamed to be your daughter.'

'That's enough,' Harry barked. 'I'm still your father and the head of this house. Watch your tongue!'

Errol sniggered and threw his cigarette into the sink. 'You're not my father, though, are you, *Uncle* Harry?'

'Of course I am. I don't know what twaddle my mother has been spouting, but I'm your father and that's an end to it.'

'No, I don't believe you. And look at her,' Errol said, pointing towards Carmen. 'It's written all over her face. She knows full well that you're not my dad.'

Harry glanced at his wife who looked pan-faced.

Errol lit another cigarette and blew smoke rings into the air. 'I play cards for a living,' he said. 'I can read people like an open book. Tell him the truth, *Mother*. Tell him that he ain't my dad.'

Carmen stared ahead. Her silence spoke volumes.

Errol walked back towards the kitchen door. 'See, I knew it. She's had you duped all these years too but you're too bleedin' spineless to stand up to her. I've had it with the pair of you. See ya.'

Harry heard his son's heavy footsteps thumping up the stairs. He guessed that Errol had gone to collect his belongings. Good, he'd be glad to see the back of him and at least he'd now be able to relax in his own home. But had Errol been right? Did Carmen *know* that Errol wasn't his son?

'See what you've done!' Cheryl shouted. 'You've split up

this family with your lies. I'm going too. I can't stay here, I'm too disgusted with you both.'

At last, Carmen spoke. 'Harry, stop her. She's not leaving this house.'

Harry locked eyes with his daughter and knew he wouldn't be able to prevent her from leaving. She had that same determined look on her face that he'd first seen when she'd been knee high to a grasshopper and had wanted to put on her own shoes. 'Where are you going?' he asked weakly.

'To live with my gran,' Cheryl answered defiantly. She threw them both a disdainful look and stamped from the room and up the stairs.

Harry hung his head in his hands in despair.

'You handled that well,' Carmen said sarcastically.

Harry lifted his head and looked accusingly at his wife. 'Is Errol my son?' he asked, but he already knew the answer.

Carmen didn't reply. She didn't need to. All these years, on his wife's word, he'd been lied to and had raised his brother's child. Wilf's son. But in reality, he'd always known the truth. He'd ignored his doubts and had been happy to believe Carmen. Blinded by love at the time, he supposed. But Harry had never had the same feelings for Errol that he held for Cheryl. He realised that he'd known all along that he wasn't Errol's dad. He couldn't blame Carmen. They'd concocted their web of lies together. But now they were facing the consequences of their deceptions. He wasn't bothered about Errol walking out. But it broke his heart to lose Cheryl. Would his daughter ever forgive him? He hoped so, but knowing how strong-willed Cheryl could be, he doubted it very much.

13

On Saturday morning, Winnie darted around preparing the final touches for Jan's and Terry's engagement party. She'd dug out some of the Christmas decorations and had hung paper chains across the ceiling. Standing back behind the bar, Winnie perused her efforts and decided that her pub looked very cheerful. They needed this. Everyone had been adversely affected by the Germans' nightly bombings. A good party would help to lift morale.

'Oh, Win, you've done a smashing job,' Rachel said admiringly when she came through to the pub.

'I'm rather pleased with it, even if I do say so myself. Where's Martha?'

'She's upstairs, sound asleep. I thought I'd see if you're ready to bring the food down?'

'Don't worry, love, me and Lucy can manage. You go and get yourself dolled up. It's been ages since you've worn any lippy or a nice party dress. Go on, no dawdling. I want you looking your best.'

Rachel smiled warmly and Winnie could see a light of excitement in her eyes. It was about time that the girl had something to look forward to. Winnie was determined that the party would lift everyone's spirits.

She followed Rachel upstairs and went into the kitchen, calling to Lucy. When Lucy appeared in the room, Winnie gasped at the sight of her. 'What on earth are you wearing?' she asked in shock.

Lucy's ample breasts spilled out over the neckline of her bright orange dress. And her make-up looked like it had been spread on her face with a trowel.

'Is it too much?' Lucy asked. 'I wasn't sure.'

Winnie, not known for her diplomacy, spluttered, 'You look like a prostitute!'

Lucy yanked self-consciously at her dress in an attempt to cover some of her flesh. 'I'll – erm – get changed.'

'Yes, I would. And while you're there, scrape off some of that muck on your face. You're ever such a pretty girl, love; you don't need to wear your make-up so heavily.'

Lucy scampered away leaving Winnie shaking her head in bewilderment. She looked down at her own dress. The red one that Brian had bought for her at Christmas. It hugged in all the wrong places and emphasised her large belly. Brian would have detested it but Winnie had worn it once before in spite of him. Now she thought that she should probably change too.

Ten minutes later, in a more flattering mauve dress, Winnie began to carry platters of party food downstairs.

'Is this better?' Lucy asked from the top of the stairs.

Winnie, standing at the bottom with a plate of sandwiches in one hand and a plate of sausage rolls in the other, turned to look. She smiled at Lucy. 'Oh, love, you look as pretty as a picture,' she said, admiring her sweetheart-neck black-and-pink floral dress with a silk pink flower in her hair.

'Thanks. I'll fetch some food,' Lucy replied cheerily. She skipped off towards the kitchen.

Winnie had pushed several tables together along the back wall of the pub and had covered them with white sheets. She placed the plates on the tables and Lucy brought down two more. The party wasn't due to start for half an hour but someone knocked on the door. Lucy opened it and Piano Pete ambled in.

'Hello, Winnie. Shall I start with the *Wedding March*?' he asked as he sat on the piano stool.

'No, love, it's an engagement. I should start with knocking out "Daisy, Daisy". But hold your horses, there's no one here yet.'

'I didn't want to be late. "Daisy, Daisy" is a good shout, Winnie. I'll play it as soon as the happy couple come through the doors.'

Another knock on the door followed and this time Winnie opened it to see Len standing there. He removed his flat cap as he came through.

'I shan't be stopping,' Len said. 'I've just come by to drop this off for Jan and Terry.' He held out a small package wrapped in newspaper. 'It's not much, just my old Touch Wud Charm that Renee gave me before I went off to fight during the Great War. She said it would bring me luck and it did. I reckon Jan and Terry could do with a bit of luck to start 'em off, so there you are.'

'Aw, Len, how thoughtful, thank you. I'm sure they will treasure it. Can't you stay and give it to them yourself?'

'No, Win, my Renee ain't feeling too clever today. I'd best get back home to her.'

'Hang on, don't rush off. I'll wrap you up a few sandwiches and that.'

Whilst Winnie prepared a small parcel of party food for Len to take home, Rachel came downstairs.

'You look lovely,' Lucy gushed.

Winnie turned around to see Rachel doing a quick twirl. Her dark pink dress swished up and out, showing off her shapely legs. 'That's better,' Winnie said. 'It's about time we saw you looking like your old self. What do you reckon, Len? I've got the prettiest barmaids in Battersea, eh?'

'They'll do,' Len agreed in his usual miserable manner. He thanked Winnie for the food parcel and then headed off.

'You may as well leave the doors unlocked,' Winnie told Lucy. 'People will be arriving soon.' Excitement flooded through her. She couldn't wait to see Jan's face when she walked in and saw how joyous the pub looked. And then something struck Winnie; she hadn't thought about David for the past hour. Normally, he was continually on her mind. It felt refreshing to have a break from worrying about him for a change.

Hilda came in next. 'Hello. I thought I'd get here early to lend a hand,' she said as she removed her coat.

'Thanks, love, but I think we've got it all under control,' Winnie said proudly.

'You can go upstairs and check on your granddaughter, if you like?' Rachel suggested.

'Actually, if it's all right with you, I'll probably stay up there with her for most of the time.'

Winnie, reading between the lines, guessed that Hilda must

159

be struggling with her demons. 'That'll be perfect, Hilda. Rachel can relax and enjoy herself for a few hours. I'll come up with you for a minute; I need to change my shoes. As glam as these heels are, they're killing me feet.'

Once they were in the front room, Winnie quietly asked, 'Are you coping all right?'

'Yes and no. I'm keeping busy during the day with the voluntary service but I'm not going to lie, Win, the nights are long and I'm terrified. If ever I've wanted a large whisky, it's now more than ever.'

'You're doing really well, Hilda. Look, between you and me, Rachel has been worried that, with Jan away, you'll turn back to the booze. I've told her that you won't. I hope you're not going to let her down.'

'No, I promise I won't. But it's hard. I'm struggling but I'm determined to keep off the hard stuff, for Martha's sake as much as me own. But if it's all the same to you, I'll stay up here, away from temptation.'

'You know you're always more than welcome up here, and by the way, I think you're doing marvellously. Help yourself to anything in the kitchen. I'll see you later.'

After changing her shoes for her 'old faithfuls', when Winnie went back down to the pub, she was pleasantly surprised to see that half a dozen more guests had arrived early. She couldn't be happier. The Battersea Tavern was about to throw the best party Battersea had seen in a very long time.

'I'm nearly done and then you can look in the mirror,' Cheryl told Yvonne as she finished applying a bit of lipstick to her friend's face. Cheryl had spent the past half-hour putting make-up on Yvonne and another half-hour styling her hair.

She'd hardly had any time to get ready herself. 'There you go, done,' Cheryl said, standing back to admire her work.

'Can I look now?'

'Yes, go on. You look beautiful.'

Yvonne tentatively pushed herself up off her bed and walked towards the mirror on her dressing table. Cheryl sat smiling, looking forward to seeing Yvonne's face when she saw herself.

'Is that really me?' Yvonne asked, surprised, as she gently touched her face.

'Yep. Do you like what I've done?'

'Yes, thanks, Cheryl, I love it! I wish you could make me look like this every day but I'm hardly going to see you when you move to Balham.'

'Yes, you will. I'll come and visit you every weekend and you can come to Balham.'

'I know, but it won't be the same as working with you every day. I'll miss you.'

Cheryl smiled wanly. She would miss Yvonne too. And her job at the factory. But it was too far to travel from Balham to Battersea every day for work. She'd have to find herself a local job. 'Don't start blubbering again, you'll smudge your mascara,' Cheryl warned.

Ten minutes later, the young women said goodbye to Yvonne's mum and headed for the Battersea Tavern with Cheryl lugging her suitcase. 'I hope my dad's not going to be there,' she moaned.

'That would be awkward.'

'Oh well, if he is, he is. I'll just ignore him. Come on, let's run. It's starting to spit down; we don't want your fancy hairdo ruined.'

By the time they arrived at the pub, Cheryl was breathless and relieved to be able to unburden herself of the weight of her suitcase.

'Hello, girls, you both look lovely!' Winnie exclaimed as they came through the door. 'What's with the case?' she pried.

'Oh, I've left home, Mrs Berry. Is it all right if I put this out the back until the party is finished?'

'Yes, love, of course. Ask Rachel to pop it in the kitchen.'

Cheryl handed her suitcase to Rachel and quickly scanned the pub. Thankfully, there was no sign of her father. She spotted Errol at the bar, casually leaning on it with Stephanie Reynolds draped over him. Cheryl had no doubt that the woman was keeping Errol close, guarding her territory from all the young and pretty women around. But Stephanie had no need to worry. Cheryl had got the impression from her brother that he was quite taken with her. She ambled up to them, dragging Yvonne along with her. 'Wotcha. Are you going to buy me and Yvonne a drink?' she asked Errol cheekily, ignoring Stephanie.

'What do you want, lemonade?'

'Yes, please, with a drop of gin.'

Errol turned to Lucy behind the bar. 'Two lemonades,' he said, and he smiled at Cheryl.

'With gin,' Cheryl added.

'Without gin,' Errol said.

'Oh, go on. Just one.'

'No. You're not drinking. How are you getting over to Gran's later?'

'I'll get the bus.'

'All right, but don't leave too late. I don't want you out and about during blackout.'

Cheryl nodded and picked up their drinks. 'Thanks,' she said and walked off. She didn't want to hang around her older brother with him watching her every move and nagging at her like her father. Today was about having fun and enjoying herself. She sashayed towards a table near the door. 'We'll sit here and wait for Carol and Anne. It's a good spot; we can see if any nice-looking fellas come in.'

Yvonne was still blushing from their encounter with Errol and Cheryl noticed that her friend's eyes kept flicking back over to the bar where he stood. She wished Yvonne would give up carrying a torch for Errol and hoped that they'd meet a couple of nice men today. As the pub began to fill with people, Cheryl thought it was looking hopeful.

She was about to make her way back to Errol and to ask him for another drink, but then Bernie came flying through the door, announcing, 'They're here!', so Cheryl remained seated. Piano Pete began playing a familiar tune and everyone looked towards the door. Moments later, a loud cheer erupted when Jan and Terry walked in. Jan looked quite flustered at the fuss and tears welled in her eyes as she stretched out her arms towards Mrs Berry.

'Thank you, thank you so much,' Jan gushed, tenderly embracing her adoptive mother.

Cheryl felt a pang of jealousy. Her own mum would never cuddle her like Mrs Berry did Jan. And Jan wasn't even Mrs Berry's real daughter. *Sod her mother*, Cheryl thought, her lips pouting and her eyes downcast as she pictured her mum's sour face.

'They look happy,' Yvonne said, breaking into Cheryl's bitter thoughts.

'Yes, they do,' she agreed. 'I'll get us another drink from Errol. You stay there and hold the table. It's getting really busy in here now.'

The party was in full swing when Carol and Anne turned up. They went to the bar, and then joined Cheryl at the table. 'Better late than never,' Cheryl said to them over the sound of the piano and people singing along.

'We would have been here sooner but Anne's sister turned up and asked us to watch her kids while she went to queue at the coal yard. Anyway, it looks like a smashing party.'

'It is but I haven't spotted any eligible young men, just all the usual faces.'

'Oh well, I suppose that's to be expected in here. Is that your brother at the bar?'

'Yes. With Stephanie flamin' Reynolds.'

'Well, it's probably a good job that there's no fellas trying to chat you up. Your Errol would scare 'em off,' Carol laughed.

Mrs Berry came over to the table with a tray of drinks. 'I'll expect you to be polite to my staff,' she warned Carol as she placed the glasses on the table. 'Help yourselves to food. There's plenty there.'

Carol nodded.

When Mrs Berry was out of earshot, Carol leaned forward. 'I think I saw Lucy with Mrs Berry's son the other day. They were coming out of the park. I was on the bus so I couldn't get a proper look but I'm sure it was them.'

'Are you going to tell Mrs Berry?' Cheryl asked.

'No, it's none of my business and I don't think she'll thank me for stirring up trouble. I've already warned her about Lucy. It's up to them.'

'Yes, it's probably best that you stay out of it. But I wonder if David knows what he's getting himself into?'

'Gawd knows. And Lucy must know what he's like. It's common knowledge that he left Rachel with the baby. Lucy is as much as a fool as he is. Good luck to 'em, they deserve each other.'

Cheryl glanced behind towards Lucy. She saw her discreetly watching Errol and wondered if Lucy fancied him. Cheryl suspected that if Stephanie wasn't stuck to Errol like baby poop to a nappy, then Errol might flirt with Lucy. She looked his sort. Slim, blonde and pretty. But having learned from Carol about Lucy's history with men, Cheryl was pleased that her brother had a possessive girlfriend. Even Stephanie Reynolds was a better choice of girlfriend than the loony Lucy Little.

Each time the door to the pub opened, Lucy felt her heart thud. But so far, David hadn't walked in. She hadn't seen him since she'd been late arriving at the park and he'd gone, despite her efforts to track down where he was staying. Now she had a strong suspicion that he'd turn up today. She hoped so but she also dreaded how Winnie and Rachel would react to him. She thought how lovely it would be if they welcomed him but she knew that would never happen. Poor David, she thought, feeling sorrier than ever for him. All around, the customers, friends and families were celebrating, yet David, Winnie's own flesh and blood, was considered an outcast.

Lucy, deep in thought, was startled by Winnie's sharp voice beside her.

'Come on, what are you just standing there for? There's folk want serving, missy. Honestly, you're like a fart in a colander today.'

'S-sorry,' Lucy stuttered, stupidly worried that Winnie would guess who she'd been thinking about. As she turned to walk to the other end of the bar, she heard Winnie's voice again.

'Oh no, for Christ's sake. What's he doing here, today of all days?'

Instantly, Lucy knew that David had walked in. Her pulse raced as she spun around to look towards the door. When she saw him standing there and looking directly at her, she felt quite giddy and, for a moment, Lucy thought that she might faint.

Winnie marched from behind the bar, rolling her sleeves up as she went. The pub had fallen deathly quiet. Even Piano Pete had stopped playing and was sitting on his stool with a roll-up stuck on his bottom lip as he stared at David.

'Oh, no you don't, not today,' Winnie said gravely to her son. 'You're not spoiling the party. OUT. NOW. You're not welcome here.' She pointed to the door behind him.

Lucy swallowed hard. She wanted to run into David's arms and beg Winnie to forgive him. Rachel appeared beside her. 'I'm going upstairs,' she whispered.

Lucy nodded but kept her eyes fixed on David, wondering if he would cause a scene or leave quietly.

'I just wanted to give the happy couple my best wishes,' David said. 'After all, it's not every day that my *sister* gets engaged.'

'Right, you've done that, so now you can leave.'

'Aren't you even going to offer me a drink?'

'You've been told, Son,' Bill warned and he stepped towards David. 'You're not welcome. Your mother has asked you to leave so I would strongly suggest that you do.'

David eyed Bill from head to foot. 'Who do you think you are, telling me what to do? And I'm not your *son*.'

Lucy tensed. She hadn't wanted David to become confrontational. If he caused trouble, it would play straight into the witches' hands. But before anyone else could speak, the air-raid siren screamed out.

'Saved by the bell,' Bill said, shaking his head in disgust at David.

'I don't believe this,' Winnie moaned. Then she shouted, 'They're early today. Sorry, folks, the party is over. Can you make your way to your homes and shelters as quickly and as safely as possible, please?'

David didn't move. He stood on the spot as Winnie ushered her customers out of the door. Some ran, some meandered, some looked petrified, while others appeared calm. Cheryl and Yvonne dashed from their table and over to Winnie.

'We've got nowhere to go,' Cheryl blurted. 'I can't go home and Yvonne's mum doesn't have a shelter.'

'All right, calm down. You can stop in my cellar. Go with Jan and Terry. Take plenty of food down with you. I don't want to see it going to waste.'

'I'll wait for you, Win,' Terry said and stood by Winnie's side, staring intimidatingly at David.

Rachel appeared again, now with Martha in her arms and Hilda behind her. 'Come on,' she told Lucy urgently. 'Let's get downstairs.'

Lucy stood firm, still watching David. As the small crowd of revellers left the pub, she saw David throw her a smile and then he turned on his heel and he left too. In all the commotion, Winnie hadn't seemed to notice and was looking behind the bar for the door key. Lucy quickly peered around her. There seemed to be a quiet panic in the air. As the pub emptied, hoping to be overlooked, she dashed through the door too and out onto the street.

The low sun in the sky was dazzling, but she saw David walking towards the corner shop and hurried after him, calling his name. When he turned around and saw her running in his direction, he opened his arms to greet her. Lucy readily fell into them. 'I didn't know if I was ever going to see you again,' she cooed, resting her head against his chest, her arms wrapped around his waist.

'Won't my mother wonder where you are?'

'I don't care. I had to be with you.'

The low and distant rumble of plane engines hedged closer. They could hear the distinctive sound of the anti-aircraft guns firing shells into the sky. The street had cleared now. Everyone, apart from them, had taken cover.

'We'd better find somewhere safe,' David said. He took Lucy's hand and pulled her along, past the shop and towards the main road.

'Where are we going?' Lucy asked. The planes were over-head now. She screamed and stopped running, ducking with her hand over her head as the sound of a nearby explosion vibrated through the air.

'We can go to my mate's house. There's a shelter there. Hurry, they're getting closer.'

Lucy, still gripping David's hand, ran as fast as she could. She dared not look up but she could hear the German fighter planes fighting with the British defence. The ground shook as another explosion thudded and then boomed with a deafening noise. 'We're not going to make it,' she cried.

A thick plume of black smoke and dust billowed out from behind the top of the houses on the next street. The smell of burning twitched her nostrils. Another loud explosion made her scream again. 'David! David!' she cried. Shrapnel from the planes fighting overhead rained down around them. Incendiaries whistled through the air, plummeting from the sky and igniting the roofs of houses. The thickening smoke from the fires blotted out the daylight. Lucy had never been so frightened for her life.

Two air-raid wardens ran towards them, both carrying stirrup pumps to extinguish the small fires caused by the incendiary bombs. 'You need to take cover,' one of them yelled at David. 'Get that woman to safety, right now!'

'I am,' he shouted back, before dragging Lucy up a narrow alley between two houses.

'In here,' David said and he pulled her through a back-garden gate. She saw a large mound of mud and dirt and, underneath, the welcome sight of the door to an Anderson shelter.

David yanked it open while Lucy covered her ears to the sound of a woman screaming in pain somewhere close by. There were more explosions, this time three or four in a row. Everything seemed to rattle. For a moment, Lucy wasn't sure where she was. It felt as if she was in the middle of a nightmare, trapped in hell. Fires burned, houses lay flat and destroyed, smoke filled the air; there was gunfire from above, the terrific sound of the bombs, the planes, the screaming. It was too much!

'Get in,' David yelled, pushing her roughly through the door.

Inside the small space, the calm contrast to outside brought Lucy to her senses. As her eyes adjusted to the dim light, she saw four shocked faces staring at her.

'It's bad out there,' David said. 'This is Lucy. Hello, Mrs Skinner.'

'Come in, come in,' Mrs Skinner beckoned, and she told her three children to shift up and make space.

The shelter was cramped and smelt awful but Lucy was grateful to be away from the horrors outside, though she still didn't believe that they weren't about to be killed.

Mrs Skinner poured Lucy a cup of black tea from a flask. 'It's not much but it'll have to do,' she said as she handed her the cup. 'Is my house still standing?'

Lucy took the cup in her shaking hand but found she was unable to speak. Instead, she nodded her head. Several larger explosions ensued, rattling the Anderson. Dirt fell in through the joints and two of the children huddled together in tears, crying softly into each other.

'We'll be all right, it'll be over soon,' Mrs Skinner soothed.

'I can't believe they've hit Battersea so badly again,' David mumbled.

'Well, the Jerries bombed Buckingham Palace. What's good enough for His Majesty is good enough for us,' Mrs Skinner said and tutted.

Lucy glanced at David. He was brushing brick dust from his dark hair. It had been a miracle that they had survived but it wasn't over yet. The shelter shook again and Lucy gasped as they heard the muffled sound of falling debris landing on top of them. She wanted to cry too but she had to try and be strong for the sake of the children. She looked down into her tepid tea, silently praying that her mum and siblings were safe. Battersea had been stuck hard and the bombs were still falling. Lucy had an awful feeling that life was never going to be the same again.

Winnie shook her head. 'Where on earth has that girl got to?' she wondered out loud.

'The last time I saw her, she was standing behind the bar. I assumed she was following me and Hilda down here,' Rachel answered.

'I didn't notice,' Jan said quietly.

'I think she may have gone after David,' Cheryl offered.

'What? Why would she do that?' Winnie asked in disbelief. Then her suspicions rose. 'Is there something you're not telling me?' she asked Cheryl.

The girl stepped from one foot to the other, looking uncomfortable.

'Out with it,' Winnie demanded.

'I don't know, Mrs Berry. Just something that Carol mentioned earlier. She told me that she thought she saw Lucy with David the other day, coming out of the park together.'

Winnie slumped back into the deckchair, her mind turning. If Lucy was secretly seeing David, then it would explain her cagey behaviour.

'Huh, I don't believe it, what's wrong with her!' Rachel exclaimed. 'There was us thinking that she was seeing a married man and, all the while, she's been sneaking about behind our backs seeing *him*.'

'Well, she might not be. Carol couldn't be sure it was them. She only *thought* it might have been,' Cheryl said.

'No, it was them, I know it,' Rachel snapped. Then, after a slight pause, she jumped to her feet and cried, 'I bet she's taken Martha to see him!'

Winnie huffed and puffed as she tried to push herself forward in the deckchair. She wished she hadn't sat in the bloody thing now. 'Slow down, love, you don't know that for a fact.'

'I do. Think about it, Win. She kept on at me about taking Martha out. Now it all makes sense. Christ, I'm so angry with her, I could kill her.'

'I'm sorry,' Cheryl muttered, 'I shouldn't have said anything.'

'I would have been disappointed with you if you hadn't,' Winnie said. 'But I'll thank you girls to keep whatever you hear down here to yourselves, please.'

Cheryl and Yvonne nodded in unison. Though Winnie suspected that the conversation would be relayed to at least Carol and Anne and she feared the whole factory would soon know all their business.

Rachel had sat back down again. Winnie could see that her brow was furrowed in deep thought and she had a good idea what was going through the girl's mind. 'Don't worry, love. She'll have to go. We can't have her living here with us anymore.'

'I couldn't bear the thought of her being here, Win. What if her and David were planning on stealing Martha?'

'I shouldn't think they would do anything like that. But I'll pack her stuff and leave it outside. Better to be safe rather than sorry, eh.'

'Thanks, Win.'

'Well, some bloomin' engagement party this is!' Winnie said with a forced chuckle.

'It's been smashing, thanks, Winnie,' Terry said and he placed his arm across Jan's shoulders.

'I should be at the hospital,' Jan said quietly. 'I'll be needed.'

The terrifying noise of bombs destroying parts of Battersea were muted in the cellar but Winnie knew that there was devastation outside. And it wasn't safe for Jan to be making her way to the hospital. 'Yes, love, you will be needed. But you can't go anywhere tonight. I suggest you make yourself as comfortable as you can and try and get some rest, then you'll be in better form tomorrow for work. And they'll still need you there tomorrow, just as much as they do now.'

'Yes, you're right.'

'Now then,' Winnie said and she turned her attention to Cheryl. 'What's all this about you leaving home? I'm sure your father won't be happy with that.'

Cheryl bristled. 'I don't care. I'm moving in with my gran in Balham.'

'I see. What about your job?'

'I'll get a new one.'

'Aw, poor Yvonne. You'll miss her, won't you, love?'

'Yes, I really will,' Yvonne answered.

Winnie wracked her brains for something else to say. For anything to fill the void of silence that was punctuated with the noise of bombs landing, possibly on their friends and families. No one had said anything, but Winnie knew that Yvonne must be worried sick about her mum, and Cheryl about her parents. And all the while, as the bombs fell around them and Winnie tried to keep up their cheer, she was secretly scared for David's life too.

14

Carmen had managed to get some sleep but Harry had been awake all night. He'd lain on the camp bed listening to every sound outside their shelter. And now, as the all-clear sounded, he was dreading opening the door, sure that they would discover their house had been flattened.

Carmen's eyes fluttered open and she sat, looking over at Harry with a deeply worried expression on her face. He wanted to tell her that everything was fine, but he couldn't. Earlier, when a loud whoosh had seemed to suck all the air from the shelter, followed by an almighty loud thump and shaking, Harry had known that the bomb had exploded close by. Close enough for it to have landed on their house. He supposed he should be grateful that it had missed the shelter, but it didn't lessen the sinking feeling he had.

Harry tentatively pushed the door open and stooped to pop his head through. Even though he'd been expecting to see his house gone, the sight of seeing just a chimney breast still standing took his breath away.

'Well?' Carmen asked from behind.

Harry couldn't find the words to tell her. He pushed the

door open further and stepped into the garden; his eyes fixed on the ruined remains of their home.

'Oh, my God,' Carmen cried.

Harry watched as his wife stumbled over fallen bricks and rubble. She seemed to be aimlessly searching for any of their belongings that remained intact.

'You're wasting your time,' he told her.

'My home … my home … my beautiful home … my curtains. Where are my curtains? I have to find my curtains,' Carmen cried. She was standing on a pile of debris, her eyes filled with despair. 'They're gone. My curtains are gone! Oh, Harry, there's nothing left of my curtains! What are we going to do?' she asked, tugging at her hair.

Harry beckoned her towards him. 'Come on, sweetheart. There's nothing left. I'll get you new things, better things. And new curtains. Just thank Gawd we're alive, eh?'

Carmen accepted Harry's hand as he helped her clamber over the ruins and she stood beside him. Together, in silence, they gazed at what had been their home for most of their married life. Gone, in the blink of an eye. But now the reality was beginning to set in and Harry realised he needed to find them somewhere else to stay. The only family they had was his mother but moving in with her was out of the question. And he couldn't see any of their neighbours lending a helping hand. After all, why should they? Most of them disliked Carmen because of her haughty ways. He could only think of one person to turn to. 'Let's see if we can get a cup of tea at the pub,' he suggested.

He expected Carmen to protest but, to his surprise, she agreed. With one final glance back at the house, they headed off and Carmen suddenly gasped. 'The children – Cheryl and Errol – oh, God, Harry, are my kids alive?'

'They'll be fine, but let's get settled and then I'll look for them,' he assured her.

Carmen's shoulders were slumped as they trudged towards the Battersea Tavern. Losing the house had clearly broken her heart. Their home had been his wife's pride and joy. She'd hardly left it except to go shopping. Now that Errol and Cheryl had moved out, Harry imagined his wife must feel that she had nothing left. 'I'll make things better, sweetheart, I promise.'

Carmen didn't answer. Harry thought that maybe she was in shock. Or perhaps she felt ashamed of the fact that they were going to need help from the likes of Winnie Berry. His wife was a proud woman and would hate to rely on the kindness of others. But they had no choice and Carmen would simply have to lump it. He hoped she would at least show some gratitude.

As they made their way through the streets, Harry felt numb at the sight of devastation all around. Street after street, there were three, four or five houses, all gone, just like theirs. Fires raged as volunteer firemen fought the blazes. Children wandered around, looking shocked and dazed, some wearing gas masks. That was something to be grateful for, Harry thought; the Germans hadn't attacked with chemicals. Well, not yet anyway.

The door to the Battersea Tavern was open and inside looked busy. Rachel and Hilda were passing cups of tea around and Winnie was wrapping a sheet torn into strips around Bernie's head.

'Come on, love,' Harry said to Carmen and gently he led her towards the bar.

Cheryl walked through from out the back, carrying the suitcase she'd left with on Friday night. She stopped on the spot when she saw them.

'Are you living here?' Harry asked.

'No, I'm on my way to my gran's. Errol has just gone to borrow a mate's car and is coming back to pick me up.'

'You've seen him then, this morning?'

'Yes. He knew I was here and came to check on me.'

'Well, I'm glad you're both OK, but I've got some bad news for you. The house, our home – it's gone, sweetheart. A bomb landed on it and there's nothing left.'

'No skin off my nose,' Cheryl said in a blasé fashion but Harry could see the shock in her eyes. 'I'll see you around,' she added.

Harry watched mournfully as his daughter walked away to meet her brother.

'Are you all right, Harry?' Rachel asked.

He turned to look at Rachel, hoping she wouldn't see the tears that had welled in his eyes. He breathed deeply before answering. 'Yes, Rachel, I'm fine, but the house is gone. Any chance of a cuppa for me and the Mrs?'

'Oh, Harry, I'm so sorry. Go and sit down on the comfy seats. I'll bring you some tea and biscuits.'

Harry ushered Carmen to a long cushioned bench seat under one of the boarded-up front windows. 'Sit yourself here, I'll be back in a jiffy.'

Carmen still said nothing and now he knew that she was in a state of shock. But he thought she'd soon be back to her scathing self after a cup of strong, sweet tea. Then, Gawd help them all.

Winnie had finished bandaging Bernie's head and now she

stood with her hands on her wide hips looking around the organised chaos in her pub. When her eyes fell on Harry, she beamed broadly.

Harry walked over and had the urge to throw his arms around her. He knew he'd find comfort from her and that she'd tell him that everything would be all right. But, of course, he couldn't hold Winnie, not in the middle of a hectic pub with his wife sitting close by. 'Me house is gone, Winnie,' he said with a shrug of his shoulders.

Winnie's smile instantly vanished and she looked at him with sympathy. 'Oh, blimey, I'm sorry, Harry. But you and Carmen are both fine?'

'Yes, thanks. How that shelter stood up to a blast so close by is beyond me, but yeah, me and Carmen haven't been hurt. We're just homeless.'

'Haven't you got any family or friends who could put you up? I know most places are tight for space but people are making do on front-room floors and all sorts. What about Cheryl's gran? She mentioned that she was going to stay with her. Couldn't you and Carmen stay there too?'

'No, Winnie, it's a long story but there's no one. I'll have to see if I can find a B and B or something, but money's going to be tight. All my stock was in the house.'

'Blinkin' 'eck! There's only one thing for it. You'll have to stay here.'

'Thanks, Winnie, it's kind of you to offer, but I wouldn't want to put you out.'

'Don't be daft. I could do with a bloke around. You and Carmen can have my room. It's separate beds, mind.'

'What about you? If we have your room, where will you sleep?'

'Lucy won't be returning so I'll move into her room. See, it's no problem.'

'Are you sure?'

'I insist.'

'Thanks, Winnie, I don't know what to say.'

'You just did. Thanks is good enough.'

'You're a good woman, Winnie, the best.' Harry smiled tenderly at her and he noticed that she'd turned flame red. He hadn't meant to embarrass her with his compliment. Quickly changing the subject, he asked, 'What's happened with Lucy?'

Winnie stepped closer and lowered her voice. 'Your Cheryl told me that one of her friends saw David and Lucy together. The sly little cow is up to no good.'

'Oh, if she's been seeing David, then I can see why you don't want her here. And she never said a word to you about it?'

'Nope, not a dicky bird. I don't know, I might have thought differently if she'd been open with me and told me the truth. At least I could have warned her off him. But I don't like the fact that she's been deceitful.'

'No, it ain't on. Are you going to pull her?'

'The moment she shows her face, I'll be throwing her out. Anyway, come on, I'll show you around upstairs.'

Harry fetched Carmen, who dragged along behind. His wife offered no comment as Winnie showed her the kitchen and bathroom and where she'd be sleeping.

'I would offer you some of my clothes but they would drown you,' Winnie said with a chuckle.

'Don't worry, Winnie, you've done more than enough for us, thank you,' Harry said. 'I'm sure Carmen can make do until she can get to the market.' He eased Carmen down onto one of the single beds. 'You have a rest, sweetheart,' he told her. 'I'll come up and check on you in an hour or two.'

Carmen didn't disagree and she lay back. Outside the bedroom, Harry whispered to Winnie, 'I think she's in shock, or something. She was really upset about her curtains. Strange.'

'Leave her be for a while. Let her brain comprehend what's happened. She'll come round. Your Cheryl was in the cellar with me all night. She was up at the crack of a sparrow's fart to help me clean up. She's a good girl. She said she was going to stay with her gran. Isn't that an option for you and Carmen?'

'No, most certainly not. It's a long story.'

'No need to explain, it's none of my business. Anyway, at least she's still got a few of her bits and will have a roof over her head. And what about Errol? Has he got somewhere to stay?'

Harry could sense that Winnie wasn't keen on the idea of him moving in too and was pleased that he could tell her that Errol had his own place. It was a blessing. Harry had no desire for Errol to be living with them and he wouldn't miss the young man either.

'Right you are. Now, if you're feeling up to it, I could do with some crates being brought up from the cellar?'

Harry readily agreed. It was the least he could do. He thought Winnie had the kindest heart of anyone he knew. He'd first been attracted to her because of her cheery smile but the more he'd come to know her, the more he'd seen of her good nature and it wasn't long before he'd found himself thinking about her all the time. Once Brian had moved out, it seemed to unleash Harry's feelings and finally he admitted to himself that he was in love with her. He'd known her for years but he'd never looked at her in that way before or fancied her. She was quite plain and a bit on the plump side for his usual tastes. But Harry had found her jovial personality attractive, her good nature shining through. Anyway, he had his *other* women to satisfy his carnal needs. He sighed, thinking that it wasn't going to be easy living under the same roof and hiding his sentiments. He felt a pang of guilt twinge his conscience. His wife was lying in a bed behind the door, upset and in shock, yet he was looking lovingly at Winnie and wishing he could scoop her into his arms. 'Tell me what crates you want brought up,' he said and swallowed hard.

Down in the cellar, Harry arched his back as he drew in a long breath and tried to take in the events of the past few hours. He was grateful that at least he and his family had been spared. But their home had gone and he was left with just the clothes he stood up in. It meant he was reliant on the kindness of friends. Oh, how things had changed, and so quickly. Harry patted the inside pocket of his jacket. He had a good wodge of money in there. Enough to buy some dodgy stock to sell on for a profit. He'd have to start again from scratch but the bit of money he had was better than nothing. It would be a hard slog, but Harry was determined he'd soon be back at the top of his game. Though for now, he'd have to stay away from his other women. They cost him a fair packet, money he could ill-afford at the moment. Again, guilt stabbed at him. The very least he could do to ease his conscience was to ensure that Carmen had a nice home to be proud of. And new curtains.

★

'I'm moving in with you,' Cheryl announced to her gran when the woman opened the front door. She held her suitcase up as proof.

'Are you indeed? I don't remember inviting you to move in with me. You'd better come in,' her gran said with a smile.

In the passageway, her gran pointed up the stairs. 'Your room is the back bedroom. You can take your case up and get unpacked. I'll put the kettle on.'

Cheryl was relieved that her gran had welcomed her, especially as she didn't have a home to go back to even if she wanted to. When she opened the door to the back room, she was pleased to find it was larger than her old bedroom and pleasantly decorated. This would do very nicely, she thought, as she placed her suitcase on the peach candlewick bed cover. Eager to get back downstairs to see her gran, she left her unpacking to do later and threw her coat and hat on top of her case.

'That was quick,' her gran said. 'The kettle hasn't even boiled yet.'

'I'll hang my clothes up later. I wanted to see you. Are you all right? There's a lot of damage nearby.'

'Of course I'm all right. I'm standing 'ere, ain't I?'

'Ha, yes, that was a silly question. I spent the night in a pub cellar, Gran. It was better than the smelly Anderson at home. But it was shocking coming here this morning. Loads of Battersea has been flattened.'

'I assume your mother and father are all right?'

'Yes, they're fine, but the house has gone.'

'Oh, blimey. So that's why you've come here?'

'No, I had already moved out and was coming anyway. You don't mind, do you?'

'I suppose not. Doesn't look like I've got much say in the matter.' Edie smiled. 'And what about Errol, is he all right?'

'Yes, he's fine. He's got the luck of the devil. Him and his girlfriend have a flat off Westbridge Road.'

'He's living in sin?'

'Yes. It's outrageous, Gran. And his girlfriend is a right tart an' all.'

'Huh, just like your mother was. Finish this tea off and take it through. I'm going outside for my morning ablutions. Shan't be long, it's bleedin' cold out there,' Edie moaned with a shiver as she pointed to the privy in the backyard. 'And in case you've got any fancy ideas to go with your fancy clothes, let me put you straight, young lady. You'll take a bath once a week in front of the fire in the front room. The rest of the time, it's a strip wash at the kitchen sink and you'll have to boil the kettle. Bed at ten, up at six. I only have the wireless on for an hour a day but you're welcome to turn it on for longer. Does that suit you?'

'Yes, Gran, thank you. I don't care what your rules are, I'm just pleased to be here.'

Her gran gave a nod of her head, picked up a worn book from the side and shuffled out through the back door.

Cheryl poured two cups of tea and carried them through to the front room. Her gran joined her shortly. She stoked the fire and sat in the comfortable-looking armchair near the hearth, leaving Cheryl to sit in the cane chair.

'Errol dropped me off earlier. He said he'd like to meet you and is coming for tea later. Is that all right, Gran?'

'That's more than all right. I've been waiting to meet my firstborn grandson for over twenty-six years. Tell me, does he look like his father, Wilf?'

'Yes, I think he does. He's got my mum's dark hair and olive skin but he's got Wilf's features.'

A tear slipped from Edie's eye which she quickly dashed away. 'Silly old fool,' she muttered.

Cheryl sipped her tea and gazed warmly at her gran. She hadn't realised that meeting Errol would mean so much to her. She'd tried to persuade Errol to come in earlier but he'd said he was too busy and would come back later and bring Yvonne too. 'Gran, when Errol visits later, he's bringing my friend with him. You don't mind, do you?'

'Not at all. It's about time this old house had a bit of life in it. Finish your tea, you're coming with me into the kitchen. I doubt your mother ever taught you how to bake. We're going to make cakes. Lots of cakes. What's Errol's favourite?'

'I'm not sure but I like marble cake.'

Little under an hour later, Cheryl's dress was dusted with flour and the aroma of sweet treats baking in the oven filled the kitchen. Cheryl sat at the table and looked around the warm and cosy room. It felt so homely, unlike the starkness of her mother's kitchen. 'Do you know what, Gran? I think I'm going to like living here,' she said.

'Won't you miss your mum and dad?'

'I don't know. I'll miss my dad, I suppose, but me and Mum have never been close.'

'She's a hard woman to get close to.'

'Yes, she is. But I wish we had been. I always wanted my mum to be like Yvonne's mum. They're really good friends. I never had that with Mum. I'm not even sure that she loves me.'

'I don't think highly of your mother but I'm sure she loves you. A mother can't help loving her child. Even when your children disappoint you, you still love 'em. It's natural.'

'If you say so. I'll have to take your word for that.' Cheryl wanted to believe her gran but she thought back to her childhood. She couldn't remember her mother ever once giving her a cuddle or a kiss goodnight. If her mum loved her, she'd never shown it. And now, Cheryl thought, it was too late.

'I'll see you later,' David said and leaned in to tenderly kiss Lucy's waiting lips.

Lucy wanted his kiss to linger for longer than it did. When she opened her eyes, he was gazing intently at her.

'Remember what we said. Lie through your back teeth. Don't admit that you was with me,' he reminded her.

Lucy nodded in agreement. Though she wanted to shout it from the rooftops that she was in love with David, she understood it was best to keep their relationship a secret for now. After all, she didn't want to lose her job and her home. Not yet. Not when David had told her that there was something he wanted her to do first. She'd pressed him about what he meant but he'd refused to let on. He hadn't said, but Lucy guessed it was probably something to do with Martha. She wondered if David was going to ask her to take Martha and then the three of them would run away together. Lucy was thrilled at the idea but her heart hammered at the thought of stealing the baby away from Rachel. She wasn't sure if she was brave enough to go through with it but she wanted to do whatever it took to make her fella happy.

He waved her off. Lucy was reluctant to leave him and wasn't looking forward to the grilling she knew she'd receive from Winnie. But David had helped her concoct a feasible lie which Lucy felt confident Winnie would believe.

She wasn't surprised to find the Battersea Tavern open and Winnie offering tea and sympathy to her customers, but she was surprised to see how busy the place was. Crammed with folk, some injured, a few in tears and others in seemingly good spirits. Men, women and children, many would have lost their homes last night. Some might have lost loved ones too.

Lucy wove her way through the pub until she met Winnie's accusing glare from behind the bar.

'You've got some nerve,' Winnie hissed quietly.

'What? I'm sorry I wasn't here earlier, but my mum was in a right state,' Lucy lied.

'Don't give me that. Do you think I was born yesterday? You've been seeing David, haven't you?'

Lucy swallowed hard. 'No, of course I haven't. Why would you think that?'

'You've been seen with him. And you followed him out of here last night.'

'No, Winnie, that's not right. I couldn't have been seen with him, that's impossible. And I didn't follow him out of here. I ran to my mum's house. I called out to you when I left. I told you where I was going. Didn't you hear me?'

'No, I never heard you say anything about running to your mum's house.'

'Well, I shouted it loud enough but I suppose with the sound of Moaning Minnie wailing out and what have you – I'm sorry, I thought you'd heard me. And then once I got to Mum's, it got so bad and the bombs were so close that I couldn't risk coming back. I stayed the night in her shelter. It was horrible, stuck in there with my stepfather. Every time he even so much as looked at me, I shook like a leaf. All I wanted to do was get away from him and come back here. I just wanted to come home to you, Winnie,' Lucy said and she lowered her eyes as she forced tears to fall.

Winnie's voice softened. 'You're not seeing David, then?'

'No, of course not,' Lucy cried. 'I'm so glad to be home and away from that – that evil man. I swear, Winnie, he wanted to take his belt to me again. I could see the hatred in his eyes. Why? Why does he hate me so much? I've never done anything to him.' Her tears were falling freely now and Lucy could see that she'd appealed to Winnie's softer side.

'It's all right, love. Don't make a scene in front of everyone, eh? Get yourself upstairs and cleaned up. Then when you're ready, we could do with a hand down here. Oh, and by the way, Mr and Mrs Hampton have moved in. Their house was bombed.'

Lucy was pleased that she'd managed to pull the wool over Winnie's eyes but now she had to convince Rachel too. Creeping up the stairs, she could hear Rachel in the kitchen, cooing to Martha. A pang of guilt struck her and she pondered whether she really was capable of stealing the baby. But she reasoned that David had as much right to raise the child. And though Lucy knew she could never love Martha as her own, she vowed to ensure the child would never go without.

Rachel emerged from the kitchen just as Lucy reached the landing.

'What are you doing here?' Rachel asked sourly, pulling Martha closer.

'There's been a misunderstanding but I've cleared it up with Winnie.'

'You're not welcome here,' Rachel spat with contempt in her eyes.

'That's not what Winnie says. Look, I know you both thought that I've been seeing David, but I haven't. So let's just forget it and get back to normal.'

Rachel didn't seem convinced. 'Prove it,' she snapped.

'What, prove I've not been seeing David? How?'

'I don't know but I don't believe you.'

'Rachel, I swear I've had nothing to do with him. I've had an awful night crammed up with my stepdad. All I want to do is get myself a cup of tea, have a wash and then go downstairs and help Winnie. David is the last person on my mind. I never have and I never will have anything to do with him.'

'I want to believe you, Lucy, but Carol saw you with him coming out of the park.'

'I don't know what Carol saw but it wasn't me. I *never* go to the park. I had a terrible experience in the park once. A man attacked me. I've not been back there since. Look, I swear any business about me and David is just nonsense. I don't know about you, but I'm exhausted. Do you want a cuppa?'

Rachel sighed. 'I suppose so.'

Lucy smiled inwardly. She'd done it. She'd convinced Rachel too. She couldn't wait to tell David about how easily she'd fooled the witches. He would be so proud of her. And even more proud of her when she snatched Martha away and then they could start their happy life together as a family.

15

As Sunday morning slipped into Sunday afternoon, Winnie tried to make the day as normal as possible. But it wasn't easy to put on a front and pretend that everything was fine and dandy. Nothing was fine and it certainly wasn't dandy. Battersea had suffered a harsh attack by the Germans. Fires burned and bodies were still being dug out from wrecked buildings. The destruction could be smelt in the air and was etched on the sorrowful faces of her customers.

'Lucy, pop upstairs and tell Rachel to peel all the spuds we have. And the carrots too. Put the chicken on to roast and anything else that you can find. I'm sure there's some sausage meat left and some bacon too. We can't expect folk to be happy if they ain't got full bellies.'

'That's very kind of you, Winnie,' Len said from the end of the bar.

'I wish there was more I could do.'

'Tell you what, my Renee is feeling much better. I'll go home and fetch her. We can bring our Sunday roast and anything else we've got and add it to your food.'

'Aw, Len, that's a smashing idea. We all need to pull

together,' Winnie said. Then she looked around at her bruised and battered customers. Not all of them bore physical wounds but most of them had been emotionally damaged in last night's raid. Winnie rang the bell that normally signified last orders. The gentle hum of the pub quietened and everyone looked towards her. 'Some of you ain't got homes to go to. And some of you can't face going home alone right now. My Sunday roast is cooking and you're all welcome to join me. If anyone has any spare food at home that they can contribute, I'd be much obliged. Dinner will be served in a couple of hours. In the meantime, let's not let those Jerry bastards keep us down.'

Len began a slow round of applause and soon the whole pub was clapping Winnie. She felt embarrassed but was pleased that her gesture had seemed to lift the mood.

Bernie, with the bandage around his head almost covering his left eye, asked, 'Is it all right if I bring me family, Winnie? My brother and his wife and their kids too? We won't come empty-handed.'

'Of course it is, love. Go and get them.'

Harry sidled up to the bar. 'You're a good woman, Winnie,' he said and gave her one of his winks.

'I just hope the Germans don't come early again and ruin me dinner,' Winnie whispered to him which made Harry chuckle. Then she added, 'But if they do, I don't see any reason why we can't eat in the cellar, it's plenty big enough down there.'

Her customers milled in and out, some leaving to go home and collect rationed food to contribute, others to fetch their families. 'Bring plates and knives and forks too,' Winnie called.

By the time dinner was almost ready, the pub was full. 'I'm

worried there might not be enough to go round,' she said quietly to Hilda.

'You needn't worry, Win, there's enough food to feed a whole battalion of the British army. No one is going to leave here hungry. You've done a terrific job.'

Rachel and Lucy began bringing bowls of steaming veg from upstairs while Hilda carried food in from the small kitchen at the back. Bernie's wife lent a hand and Renee organised where everything was to go.

'Don't stand on ceremony,' Winnie shouted, 'get stuck in!'

Her stomach grumbled at the aroma of cooked meats and her mouth salivated at the sight of the roast potatoes. But just as she was about to fill her plate, the door flew open and Bill rushed in.

'There's a big fight in the air over Kent but heading this way,' he blurted. 'I've heard it on the wireless. Hundreds of German bombers and fighters. Spitfires and Hurricanes have been scrambled. Several planes have been shot down. But the Jerries are doing their best to get to London!'

Winnie placed her plate down and, though she was terrified and also peeved that their meal had been interrupted, she refused to allow the Germans to ruin it. 'Right, you all heard Bill. No need to panic. Men, grab some tables and chairs. Take 'em down to me cellar. Ladies, carry the plates and the food down. Lucy, find as many candles as you can in the back kitchen. Chop-chop, we don't want to be eating cold cabbage.'

There was a flurry of activity as everyone followed Winnie's instructions. A couple of young lads rushed outside to the street. One came darting back in through the door, insisting that he could see *millions* of planes in the sky. The air-raid siren began to screech, the long and monotonous low and high wail becoming a too-familiar sound to Winnie.

Hilda tapped her on the shoulder, saying, 'Winnie, come on, you can't stay up here.'

She glanced around her empty pub. How much longer could they continue to live like this? How many more men, women and children would be killed in the next few hours? The heartbreaking thought made her appetite instantly disappear. But, as always, as she turned towards the cellar door, Winnie pushed her shoulders back defiantly and plastered on a big smile.

'Gran, we can't stay in the house when the bombers come, it's not safe,' Cheryl argued.

'It's been good enough till now. I'm not budging.'

'Please, Gran. Let's go down to the underground station.'

'What would I want to do that for?'

'For me. I can't sleep in my bed thinking about a bomb landing on us.'

'You go, I'm not stopping you.'

'I can't leave you here by yourself.'

'Course you can. Anyway, the Government have made it quite clear that they don't want us using the tube stations as shelters.'

'It hasn't stopped people. I was talking to Mrs Monk next door. She said all you have to do is buy a ticket to the next stop and then just stay on the platform. The station master ain't stopping people. Mrs Monk was down there last night. She said it was jam-packed but she slept like a baby.'

'For Gawd's sake, if it shuts you up, I'll go. Cor, you don't 'alf keep on.'

'Thanks, Gran,' Cheryl said as she leapt to her feet. She leaned down to kiss her gran's cheek. 'I'll get us a flask ready and some sandwiches. You might want to take your knitting or something.'

'All this blinkin' palaver when I was quite happy in me bed. But, if it keeps you happy, madam.'

'It does, thank you. Right, now that's sorted, I'll put the kettle on for a cuppa.'

As Cheryl went to the kitchen, there was a loud hammering on the front door. Sensing the urgency, she rushed to answer it and found Mrs Monk on the step.

'My Ted has just heard on the wireless that there's a lot of planes fighting from Manston. The Germans will be trying to break away and will be making their way up the Thames Estuary soon. Ted knows about this stuff; he don't miss a trick. We're going down the tube station early. Are you and Edie coming?'

'Yes, I've managed to talk some sense into my gran. I'll just make a flask and then we'll be ready.'

'All right, but don't dawdle.'

Cheryl went back into the front room and announced gravely, 'We have to go now, Gran.'

Edie didn't hesitate and scooped up her knitting bag. She shoved two magazines inside and a newspaper.

Cheryl tapped her foot impatiently as she waited for the kettle to boil. Her mind turned as she tried to think of what they should take with them. Blankets, maybe, and pillows? Yes, that would be a good idea. If she could make her gran comfortable on the platform, then Edie might be inclined to use the shelter again. Cheryl dashed around the house grabbing what she needed. She pulled out their coats from under the stairs, then she heard the kettle whistling. Minutes later, they were outside in the sun, laden with bedding and bags.

'Let me take that for you,' Ted Monk offered, and he held out his hand for Edie's knitting bag.

'I can manage, dear,' she replied.

Together in anxious silence, they trudged the short distance down the hill to the underground train station. Cheryl was surprised to see a long queue had already formed.

'Seems everyone's got the same idea as us,' Mrs Monk remarked.

'Are you all right, Gran?' Cheryl asked.

'Yes, dear. Though I'd rather be sitting in me chair with me feet up.'

The queue slowly went down and Cheryl found herself inside the station at the ticket office. She bought a ticket for her and her gran but when she turned to the escalator, she saw that many people were rushing down the stairs without tickets and no one was bothering to stop them. Even Mr and Mrs Monk had gone through.

'Keep hold of my arm,' Cheryl instructed her gran. 'We don't want to lose each other.'

Cheryl led her down the escalator and through to the southbound platform. She was shocked to find so many people already bedded down. The platform was strewn with bodies and the stench was quite overpowering.

'I can't sleep down here with this lot,' her gran said, wrinkling her nose in disgust.

'Let's try the other platform,' Cheryl suggested. But she was sorely disappointed to find that it was even busier on that side. 'We'll go back to the other one.'

'No, it's all the same,' her gran answered. 'We may as well stay here now and make the best of it.'

A woman a few years older than Cheryl was sitting on the paved floor against the dirty tiled wall. She glanced up at Edie hobbling through the crowd and then told her young boys to get up off the bench and allow Edie to sit there.

'Thank you, thank you very much,' Cheryl mouthed to the woman.

As her gran did her utmost to make herself comfortable, much to Cheryl's surprise, a gust of wind whooshed through the tunnel followed by a train coming into the station. Passengers disembarked and made their way off the platform through a gap in the people – it was only about a yard wide.

'The trains stop running at ten-thirty,' the woman informed Cheryl. 'Earlier on a Sunday. And then as the platform overflows, the lines down there get filled up with families too.'

Cheryl had never seen anything like it. She'd hated being in the Anderson in their backyard but this was even worse. Nevertheless, she did feel safe being so far underground.

As the train left the platform and sped off through the dark tunnel, word began to spread that the air-raid siren was sounding. Cheryl looked at her gran who was pulling her knitting from her bag. 'We did the right thing by coming here early. The siren is sounding.'

'If you say so.'

Cheryl smiled inwardly. She had a lot to learn about her gran. One thing she'd already discovered was that her gran was stubborn, just like her.

★

Harry had managed to drag a reluctant Carmen from Winnie's bedroom down to the cellar. He sat her at a table and placed a plate of food in front of her.

'Eat up,' he said. 'We don't know when our next meal will be.'

He could see that Carmen's eyes were swollen from crying. She'd shed her tears in private, which Harry was relieved about. Upset women made him feel uncomfortable. But his heart went out to his wife. Her whole life had been wrapped up in their home and now everything had been blown to smithereens.

'It ain't 'alf bad, this grub, but not as good as your Sunday dinners,' he said, trying to lighten her mood.

Carmen, with her hands on her lap, stared down at the plate of food.

'Try and eat something, eh, sweetheart? It'll do you good.'

'I'm not hungry,' Carmen hissed and pushed her plate away.

'Shall I get you a hot drink? Or a glass of stout?'

Carmen ignored Harry's offer and turned her face to one side. He got the feeling that she somehow blamed him for the atrocity that had happened to their house. Or maybe she was just taking her anger out on him. He tucked into his lunch but couldn't help feeling useless.

Winnie called across the cellar, 'Have you all got enough to eat?'

A unanimous 'Yes, thanks,' resounded though the room. With all the chatter and the clinking of knives and forks on plates, it was difficult to hear the muted sounds of bombs exploding outside. But Harry could see by the expressions on people's faces that everyone knew what was going on around them. Thankfully, no one mentioned it but Harry felt scared through to his bones and assumed that most other people must be too. He'd seen first-hand the destruction that a bomb could do. And though being in the cellar offered some protection, it seemed to give them a false sense of security. If one of Hitler's explosives were to land on the Battersea Tavern, Harry knew that everyone down there would likely be killed instantly.

16

On Monday morning, Winnie woke up with her back aching. After yet another prolonged attack on London throughout the night, once they'd heard the all-clear, she'd slept for a few hours on the lumpy sofa in the front room. Her sleep had been restless and she'd spent much of the time thinking about Harry, who was sleeping just several feet away in the next room. Once again, Winnie chastised herself for having such ridiculous thoughts. But it didn't stop her checking her reflection in the mirror, something she wouldn't normally do first thing in the morning. She was sure she could hear Harry in the kitchen.

'Good morning, sweetheart,' he greeted her.

Winnie noticed that Harry's clothes appeared crumpled. She was about to offer to press his suit for him but realised that Carmen's nose might be put out of joint so, instead, she made a mental note to offer the iron to Carmen.

'The kettle has nearly boiled. I didn't wake you, did I?' he asked.

'No, of course not. I'm always up early. Is Carmen still sleeping?'

'Yes. I'm hoping that the shock of it all has worn off now and that she'll wake up her usual self. Actually, on second thoughts, maybe it would be better for all of us if she stayed in shock.'

Harry and Winnie both chortled but their laughter was cut short when Carmen walked into the kitchen.

'This is very cosy,' she quipped. 'What's so funny?'

Harry exchanged a quick, guilty glance with Winnie. 'Nothing, sweetheart,' he answered. 'Cuppa?'

'In all the years we've been married, not once have I ever known you to make a pot of tea,' Carmen scoffed, and then she turned to Winnie, adding, 'he must be showing off for your benefit.'

Winnie felt uncomfortable and didn't know where to look or what to say.

Harry seemed to sense the uneasy atmosphere and changed the subject. 'I'm not happy about you kipping on the sofa, Winnie. It's not right. Whilst we're here, you should have your own bed and I can take the sofa. That's as long as you don't mind sharing with Carmen?'

'I'm fine on the sofa, it's not a problem,' Winnie fibbed. She'd missed the comfort of her own bed but she didn't relish the notion of sharing her room with Carmen.

'No, it's not fine. I won't hear of you sleeping on that sofa for another night. I've put my foot down, so that's that,' Harry said masterfully.

Carmen sniffed incredulously at her husband's remarks but she kept her mouth shut.

'All right. But if Carmen prefers her privacy, perhaps Lucy could sleep in with me and Carmen can have Lucy's room?'

Before Carmen had a chance to say anything, Harry jumped in. 'No need for any upheaval, but thanks.'

Winnie noticed that Carmen looked at her husband with daggers in her eyes. She obviously didn't like the fact that he'd answered on her behalf and declined the offer of Lucy's room.

'I'm going to put the breakfast on. Scrambled eggs do you both?'

'Smashing, thanks, Winnie,' Harry enthused, rubbing his hands together.

'Let me help you,' Carmen offered.

'No need,' Winnie answered politely.

After whisking the eggs in a bowl, she gently stirred them as they cooked and then quickly sliced the bread before spreading it with butter. Carmen hurried over to the stove.

'You have to keep stirring the eggs,' she said, 'or they'll set like an omelette.'

Winnie went over and looked into the pan. The eggs looked perfectly fine to her. 'Thank you,' she said curtly and took the wooden spoon from Carmen. 'I can carry on from here.'

Carmen huffed and stood beside Winnie with her eyes fixed on the pan. 'They're ready now. Still wet. Harry doesn't like his eggs overcooked.'

'I'll take 'em however they come,' Harry said from the table.

Winnie dished up his and Carmen's eggs but put her own back on to cook for a while longer. 'Make the most of them,' she called over her shoulder. 'It'll be back to powdered eggs until you get your business back up and running again, Harry. By the way, I don't suppose you brought your ration books with you?'

'As a matter of fact, we did. Carmen had the forethought to pop them into her pocket before we went into the shelter.'

'It was sheer fluke that I did. I wouldn't normally,' Carmen said and then asked, 'Won't Lucy and Rachel be joining us for breakfast?'

Winnie sat at the table looking forward to her breakfast. 'They'll both be out for the count,' she answered. 'They must be shattered. Those girls didn't stop yesterday. We had folk in and out all day. Lucy and Rachel made sure everyone was looked after. Proper angels, the pair of them.'

'Yes, well, they're young and have the energy. Though I wouldn't go as far as to call them angels, especially Rachel,' Carmen said as she sprinkled more salt on her eggs.

'What's that supposed to mean?' Winnie asked.

'Nothing,' Harry answered quickly for his wife. 'She doesn't mean anything at all, do you, Carmen?'

'Well, it's no secret that Rachel is an unmarried mother. If you ask me, it's a disgrace!'

Winnie banged her knife and fork down hard on the table. She stood up, marched around to Carmen, leaned over her shoulder and snatched up her unfinished breakfast plate. 'No one asked you, so while you're under my roof, I suggest you keep your opinions to yourself, especially about Rachel and *my* granddaughter.'

'I haven't finished that,' Carmen said and she held her hand out for her plate.

'Yes, you have,' Winnie snapped. She stamped across the kitchen and scraped the remaining eggs and bread into the bin.

Carmen looked at her husband, then at Winnie, then back at Harry. When Harry didn't jump to her defence, Carmen slowly rose from the table and slunk out of the room with her nose held high in the air. Once she'd left the room and they heard the bedroom door close, Winnie and Harry both let out a long breath.

'I'm sorry about her,' Harry said.

'No need. I know what she's like but if we're to live in harmony here, she needs to learn to keep her mouth shut. I may be a lot of things, Harry, but a pushover ain't one of them. I let Brian walk all over me for years. I won't allow the likes of her to think that she can too.'

'Good on you, girl. It's only right that you should stand up for yourself. And for the record, I don't like runny eggs.'

Winnie smiled and then asked, 'Why don't you stand up to her?'

Harry ran his finger along the inside of his shirt collar as if the thing were too tight around his neck. 'I opt for the quiet life, Winnie. It's easier for me to say nothing or to agree with her.'

'I did the same with Brian but it never got me anywhere.'

'I'd better go and see if she's all right. She's probably in there sharpening her claws.'

Winnie sat back at the table and cupped her warm tea as she watched Harry leave the room. She'd got the feeling that he was hiding something and not telling her the full story. She wondered what it could be; after all, they usually spoke so easily to each other. But there had to be a reason why Harry allowed Carmen to rule over him. Whatever that reason was, it was clear that he didn't want Winnie knowing about it.

She sighed deeply. He'd had the same effect on her as always: she felt flushed and she had butterflies in her stomach. Thankfully, neither Carmen nor Harry appeared to notice.

But now that they were all living together, Winnie knew she had to get a grip of her feelings before she ended up making a complete idiot of herself.

Lucy had been pleased when the lunchtime shift had finished. She felt tired but she was also excited about meeting David. She peered at her reflection in her bedroom mirror and groaned at the sight of dark circles ringing her eyes. She tried to conceal them with a dab of foundation that she used sparingly. Cosmetics were becoming harder to come by. Hilda had said that she was using beetroot juice to tint her lips. Luckily, Lucy had a new lipstick and splurged it across her lips, hoping that the bright colour would detract from the dark circles.

'That'll have to do,' she said to herself and pouted into the mirror.

After pulling on her coat, she walked along the passageway and called out, 'I'm popping round to my mum's for a while. See you later.'

She trotted down the stairs and heard Winnie call back, 'Ta ta, love.'

Good, she thought. It seemed that there was no suspicion about her actions.

As Lucy approached Battersea Park, she spotted David meandering along a path and she picked up her pace. He had his hands stuffed into the pockets of his jacket and his collar pulled up. She supposed it must be cold but Lucy felt as though she was glowing. *It's strange the way love makes you feel*, she thought, smiling.

'Wotcha,' David greeted her, before kissing her lightly on the cheek.

His nose felt frozen against her skin. 'Have you been here long?' she asked.

'No, I just got here. Come on, let's get to the café. I need a hot drink.'

Once inside, Lucy peeled off her coat to reveal a closely fitting, purple crocheted waistcoat which she wore over a cotton blouse. She had deliberately left the top button undone to show her cleavage. She placed her coat over the back of the seat and watched David's face to gauge his reaction.

'Your – erm – button,' he said, pointing quickly towards her chest and then looking away.

'Oh, silly me,' Lucy uttered, pretending to appear coy.

She pulled her seat round to sit closer to him and then purred, 'I missed you last night.'

'Yeah, me an' all.'

'Did you? Did you really?'

'Yeah, of course.'

'I don't know how much longer I can carry on with this façade.'

'What façade?' David asked.

'All this creeping around and sneaking about behind your mum's back. I just want to be with you. It's not a crime, is it?'

'No, it's not, but my mum will think so.'

'What are we going to do? We can't continue like this and you'll be leaving soon to go back to Richmond. I can't stand it, David, I really can't.' Lucy took a handkerchief from her handbag and dabbed at her eyes, feigning tears. 'I'd do anything to be with you. Anything at all,' she said. Surely this would be the cue he needed for him to reveal what he wanted from her. And though the idea of stealing baby

Martha frightened the life out of her, she was prepared to do it for David.

'Actually, there is something you can do for me but I don't know how to say it.'

'Just ask, David, just ask.'

'Well, the truth is, I've not been entirely honest with you. See, the thing is – my place in Richmond... I rent a room in a run-down house and the landlady is a stickler for rules. She'd never allow me to bring you to my room. But the rent is cheap; I can't afford to get kicked out.'

'Oh, I see.'

'And my job with the electric board – I lost it. They had to let me go; cutbacks.'

Before Lucy could answer, a waitress came to the table to take their orders. Lucy asked for a cup of tea and a slice of sponge cake. David said he'd have the same. Once the waitress had gone, Lucy leaned towards David. 'Given your current predicament, you'd best let me get the tea and cakes for us,' she whispered.

'Thanks. But it doesn't have to be like this. I've got a solution but I'd be asking a great deal of you.'

'I've already told you; I'd do anything for you.'

'I hate to put you in this situation, but an offer has come up that could make me a very rich man. The trouble is, I need money to invest in the first place.'

'Oh, what's the offer?' Lucy asked. She'd been disappointed to hear that there was no home in Richmond waiting for her to move into and that David didn't have a job, which would mean he wouldn't be able to support their family. But it was beginning to sound like he had a plan and Lucy was keen to know more.

'It's a mate of mine in Richmond. He owns a very success-ful business, a garage, repairing motor cars and bikes. He's got two chaps working for him but one is getting on and wants a slower pace of life and the other has signed up. Larry, my mate, he's offered me a partnership for a ridiculous price. It's too good an offer to turn down.'

'I didn't know you had any mechanical experience.'

'I had my own motorbike for years and a good friend of mine was a mechanic. We were always tinkering about together under car bonnets. Anyway, I'd learn on the job and be making loads of money at the same time. But only if I can find the cash to buy into the business.'

'I haven't got any money. If I did, I'd give it to you.'

'No, I realise that, darling. But my mum does.'

'Is that why you came back? To ask her for the money?'

'Yes. I only wanted a loan. I would have paid her back within a month or two. But you saw the reception I received. There's no chance of her lending me any money.'

'I doubt she'd lend it to me either.'

'No, she wouldn't. That's why I want you to take it. I don't want to steal from her but she's raking in good profits. She won't miss a few days' worth of takings.'

Lucy gasped. 'You want me to steal the pub's takings?' she asked aghast.

'It's not that I want you to, but I *need* you to.'

This wasn't what Lucy had been expecting that David would ask of her. And in a peculiar way, stealing money from Winnie felt even more abhorrent than snatching Martha from Rachel. 'I don't know, David. It doesn't feel right.'

'Trust me, Lucy, it'll be fine. You've seen for yourself; the pub is always busy. Me mum must be making a small fortune. She'll soon cover her losses. If there was any other way—'

'But it's theft!'

'Depends how you look at it. That pub belonged to my father but I'll never see a penny from it now. Yet my so-called *sister* gets big parties thrown for her and my mother can afford to feed half of Battersea. I'm only asking you to take a fraction of what should rightfully be mine one day. And once I'm a partner in the business, I'll get us a nice house and all the things you want.'

Lucy felt relieved when the waitress appeared with their order. It gave her a minute to think. What David said made sense and stealing money couldn't be any worse than taking Martha. If it meant that they could all be together, then Lucy decided it was worth it. 'I'll do it,' she said firmly.

'That's my girl. You're a good 'un. I promise you; I'll spend the rest of my life making it up to you.'

David's words left Lucy bursting with delight. *The rest of his life*, she thought, picturing the two of them in a nice home in Richmond with David bouncing Martha on his knee and herself with an expanding stomach, their child inside.

David interrupted her thoughts. 'You'll have to take the money next Monday morning. That's when there will be the most before Mum banks it. There will be all of Friday and the weekends takings. Do you know where she keeps the money?'

'Yes, in the oven in the back kitchen.'

'Ha, she doesn't change. My mother doesn't believe in safes. Right, that's straight forward enough. You sneak down first thing, grab the cash and then I'll meet you at Clapham Junction railway station. We'll get clean away.'

'But what if she catches me?'

'She won't, not if you're careful.'

Lucy sipped her tea with her heart pounding hard and fast. She was scared but the thought of running off together to Richmond felt exhilarating. A new life with David and Martha, away from the grime of Battersea. It was everything she'd ever dreamed of but there was just one thing missing. 'If we're to live together, don't you think you should make an honest woman of me?' she asked.

David's eyes widened. Clearly he hadn't considered marriage and for a moment, Lucy's heart sank.

'Yes, I suppose I should really. There's a registry office in Richmond. We can get married there.'

Lucy quietly squealed. 'Oh, David, really? You're going to make me your wife?'

'Yes, that's what I said, wasn't it?'

It wasn't a romantic proposal but that didn't matter to her. And it wasn't important where or how they married. She wanted to be a wife and mother more than anything and, finally, her happy future was within sight. In fact, robbing Winnie and taking Martha didn't seem to be such a harrowing thought anymore, not now that she had something wonderful to look forward to.

17

After finishing work on Friday, Cheryl flopped on her gran's sofa and kicked off her shoes.

'How was your first week at work?' her gran asked.

'Not bad, thanks, but my feet are killing me. I'm used to sitting at a bench all day, not standing up behind a counter.'

'You did well to get that job in Barratts shoe shop, especially as you've had no shop experience.'

'I think the glowing reference from Mr Mullen at the factory helped. Don't get me wrong, I'm not complaining about the job, though the smell of stinky feet is a bit off-putting sometimes.'

'I think you've done very well, dear. What with sleepless nights in the tube station and planes falling out of the sky, it's not been an easy week.'

'Maybe, but we've not had it as bad as others. I just hope Errol is all right.'

'Is he coming over again this weekend?'

'Yes, and he's bringing Yvonne too. I can't wait to see her.'

'I expect you've missed her.'

'I have. The women in the shop are all right, I suppose,

but they're a bit stuck up. And old. I can't have a laugh with them like I do with Yvonne.'

'She seems like a lovely young lady.'

'She is. I'll tell you a secret but don't let on. She's sweet on Errol. Has been for years.'

Cheryl's gran chuckled. 'He is a smashing-looking boy, just like his father, Wilf.'

'Yes, he's always got girls after him. But poor Yvonne, she doesn't have a chance with him.'

'And what about you, dear? Is there a special man that you're sweet on?'

Cheryl felt herself blush and wondered if her gran had noticed. 'No, not really,' she fibbed, thinking about Bobby the Butcher.

'Yes there is, I can see your eyes twinkling. Who is he? Someone from work?'

'No, nothing like that. It's just – oh, nothing. It's nothing.'

'Your cheeks are bright red so it's obviously something. But if you don't want to tell your old gran, that's fine.'

'It's Bobby. He works in the butcher's. But I don't even know if he realises that I exist.'

'Bobby Willmore? Tall lad, dark hair, walks with a slight limp?'

Cheryl sat forward, her eyes wide. 'Yes, yes, that's him! Do you know him, Gran?'

'I've known him since the day he was born. His grand-mother was my best friend at school. She lives on the corner of the street. Bobby lives on the next street with his mum and three brothers. Two of them have gone off fighting somewhere but Bobby was turned down on account of his back. His spine was a bit curved when he was born but he's as right as rain, apart from his slight limp. Mind you, his mother thinks it's a blessing, cos it's kept him out of the army.'

'Do you know if he has a girlfriend?' Cheryl asked hopefully.

'I don't think so. Do you want me to introduce you?'

'No!' Cheryl exclaimed, mortified at the thought. 'Oh, Gran, I would die!'

'Why? You daft moo.'

'No, please, Gran. It would be too embarrassing.'

'How else are you going to meet him, then? I suppose you could register your ration book there?'

'I don't know. I'll put the kettle on,' Cheryl said, changing the subject. She wished she hadn't said anything now and hoped her gran wouldn't meddle.

'Yes, you do that, dear. And I'll have a think about how we can get Bobby to ask you on a date.'

It appeared that any hope of her gran not meddling was quickly flying out of the window. But Cheryl smiled. Already, in just one week, she felt closer to her gran then she'd ever felt to her mother. Edie was fast becoming her friend and confidant too. But she knew that she'd always wish that things had been different with her mum.

Harry's coffers were looking rosier than they had done a week ago. He'd managed to buy and sell some knocked-off goods for a handsome profit and orders were flooding in, some customers paying cash up front. Carmen had been busy looking for somewhere to live but hadn't yet found anywhere suitable. With bombs dropping daily, housing was in high demand. Harry was enjoying staying with Winnie at the Battersea Tavern. She was good company and her bright and cheerful disposition was a pleasure to be around. Unlike his wife's. Carmen had become even more mean-spirited than normal. Harry had made concessions for her. After all, it couldn't be easy for his wife to be homeless and without her kids. But Carmen's spiteful tongue had caused a couple of arguments with Winnie. He thought the woman was a saint for putting up with his wife's moods but Harry worried she wouldn't for much longer. For a fleeting moment, he wished his wife wasn't around and then he could be with Winnie. Not that he wanted Carmen dead or anything like that. He just wished she'd disappear and leave him in peace.

He walked to the kitchen doorway and glanced up and down the passageway. When no one was in sight, Harry went back to the kitchen table and sat opposite Carmen. 'You need to watch what you say, sweetheart. Winnie is a generous woman but if you keep starting rows with her, she'll throw us out.'

Carmen, her lips pursed, glared at Harry.

'I know it's tough for you and you don't like living under another woman's roof, but it won't be for much longer. Just try being a bit nicer, eh?'

'You've no idea what it's like for me,' Carmen snapped.

'Shush, keep your voice down. All right, why don't you tell me, then.'

'What's the point? You don't care. Just as long as everyone *loves* Have-it bloody Harry, then you're happy. You've never had any regard for me, stuck all hours by myself. Not to mention the blind eye I turn to where most of your money goes.'

'That's not true, sweetheart. I work the hours I do to provide you with what you want.'

'Work? Don't make me laugh! You've never done an honest day's work in your life! You swan around, in this pub and that

212

pub, cracking jokes, flirting, adoring the adoration, but work, huh, tell me another.'

'That *is* my work. I have to be friendly but I never flirt. Why would I? I've got a beautiful wife right here. There ain't a woman in Battersea who could hold a torch to you,' he lied, thinking about his feelings for Winnie.

Carmen's face remained hard and he could see that his charm wasn't working on her. She'd mentioned where he spent a lot of his money. She rarely raised the subject these days, but when she did, Harry always felt terrible. Though he reasoned that if his wife didn't want him between the sheets, he had to find his pleasures elsewhere. After all, he was a man and it was a necessity.

'Don't take me for a fool, Harry Hampton! I've heard you and Winnie whispering and laughing when you think I'm not around. I know there's something going on with you two, so don't bother denying it.'

'What?' Harry blurted. He was flabbergasted at his wife's accusation. How on earth had she worked him out?

'I've seen the way she looks at you. And how flustered she gets around you. I bet she's got a guilty conscious, that's why she's so bloody nervous.'

'I don't know what you're talking about,' Harry protested. But he was somewhat relieved that it was Winnie who was getting the blame and not himself.

'I knew that's what you'd say. You're a good liar, Harry. But it's written all over Winnie's face. I never thought I'd say this, but that fat cow ain't having my husband. We're moving out of here tomorrow, no matter what. But if I get even a sniff that I'm right about you two, I'll cut your bleedin' thingy off and slap her to Wandsworth and back.'

Harry leaned back in his seat, unsure of what to say. Carmen had made her mind up and no matter what he said, she'd be unlikely to change it. He didn't want to move out and leave Winnie but there was no other choice. In the long run, he supposed it was probably for the best. After all, he couldn't risk his wife discovering his secret feelings for Winnie.

Winnie had inadvertently heard enough and she fled downstairs, humiliated by what Carmen had said to Harry. She supposed it shouldn't have come as any shock really. After all, women were astute when it came to another female having designs on their husbands. But now all Winnie wanted was to run and hide and never have to face Harry again. But with a bar full of customers, hiding wasn't an option.

'Hello, Win. Are you all right?' Hilda asked.

'Yes, love, I'm fine,' Winnie lied.

'You look a bit upset. Are you sure you're fine?'

Winnie's eyes darted around her pub. She was pleased to see that Lucy seemed to have everything under control. She whispered to Hilda, 'Come out the back.'

Hilda, looking puzzled, followed Winnie into the downstairs kitchen. 'What's going on?'

'I don't know where to start. I feel such a fool.'

'Has this got something to do with Harry?'

Winnie's jaw dropped. 'How did you know?'

Hilda pulled out a seat at the table and sat down. 'I guessed. I've seen how your eyes light up whenever he's around.'

Winnie also pulled out a seat and slumped into it. She hung her head in her hands, wanting to kick herself. 'Is it that obvious?'

'No, I don't think so. Not to anyone else.'

'It is to Carmen,' Winnie said solemnly.

'Has she said something to you?'

'No, thank Gawd. But I just heard her and Harry talking and from what I can gather, she thinks that me and him are having an affair.'

'Oh, blimey. You're not, are you?'

Winnie's head shot up to look at Hilda. 'No, of course we're not!' she snapped. 'But it didn't sound like Carmen believed him. Oh, Hilda, I'm so ashamed. I wish the ground would open up and swallow me.'

'Be careful what you wish for. Have you seen the size of some of them holes in the ground where a bomb has landed? But seriously, don't worry. You've done nothing wrong so your conscience is clear.'

'I wish you were right but I've been an idiot. Fancy getting a crush on Harry at my age, it's bloody ridiculous.'

'No, it's not. You're not that old, Win. And with Brian gone, these things happen. You can't help who you fall in love with.'

'Love? I'm not in love with Harry!'

'Are you sure about that?'

Winnie blinked hard and fast as she tried to work out her feelings. 'No, I can't be. It's just a silly crush,' she answered.

'Who are you trying to convince? Me or yourself?'

'I – erm – I don't know, Hilda. But either way, I'm a married woman and Harry is a married man. And now Carmen knows how I feel! What am I going to do?'

'Calm down and put the kettle on for a start.'

Winnie nodded and then walked across to the sink, her mind flooded with thoughts of Harry. 'How am I ever going to look him in the eye again?'

'Just in the same way as you do every day. Nothing's changed, you haven't done anything wrong.'

'But *everything* has changed. Harry knows how I feel about him. And so does his *wife*! I heard Carmen telling Harry that they would be moving out tomorrow. I've got to be honest, tomorrow can't come soon enough for me.'

'There you go, problem solved.'

'But it's not, though, is it? I mean, Harry will still be in here every day conducting his business. And it's not like I can afford to bar him. His customers always buy a drink when they're here and I need the money more than ever. Brian is chasing me for his cut, the tax has gone up, the price of beer has increased and I've been spending money that I ain't got on tea, bandages, food and all sorts, just trying to help out those less fortunate.'

'Then you need to stop doing that, Win. You can't help the whole of Battersea. It's very commendable of you but just slow down. You're taking on too much, what with all this early morning opening for free tea and biscuits and the like. If you're not careful, you'll have people taking advantage of your good nature.'

'Yeah, maybe. But that aside, what the hell am I going to do about Harry?'

The kettle whistled and Hilda finished making the tea. Winnie told her to bring the biscuit tin over and, in usual fashion for Hilda, when she sat back down, she poured her tea from her cup into her saucer, and then gently blew on it before slurping it up. Winnie sat quietly, patiently waiting for Hilda to suggest something.

Finally, Hilda spoke and asked, 'If Harry left Carmen, would you be interested in being with him?'

'No, no, no, no, no, never. Anyway, even if I wanted to be

with him, Harry would never want to be with someone like me.'

'What are you on about? You and him get on like a house on fire. You're always laughing and joking together. It's a joy to see.'

'Yeah, we're good mates but Harry doesn't see me as anything more than that.'

'You know that for a fact, do you?'

'Well, no, but it's obvious,' Winnie replied.

'Actually, Win, I think you could be wrong. What if Harry is in love with you too?'

'Will you stop saying *in love* with. I've told you, it's just a crush. And you're barking up the wrong tree with Harry. He could never love me.'

'I think you underestimate yourself.'

'Look, all this ain't helping. I need to know how I'm going to walk back into my pub and hold my head high in front of him and Carmen.'

'That's exactly what you do. Just act as if nothing has happened. Remember, you put them up in your home, Carmen ought to be grateful. And as for Harry, well, I don't know what to say; just smile and be as normal as you can.'

Winnie sipped her tea. She'd been hoping that Hilda would have suggested something more helpful. And though Hilda hadn't intentionally done so, she'd made matters so much worse for Winnie. Not only did she have her shame and embarrassment to deal with, but now she was questioning how she felt about Harry. What may have started as just a small crush, Winnie realised had grown into something out of her control. The realisation hit her like a double-decker tram: she was madly in love with Harry Hampton and there was nothing she could do to make her feelings go away.

Once Winnie had pulled herself back together, Hilda went upstairs to see Rachel and Winnie went back through to her pub. At the same time, Bill walked in. It was no surprise to see him on a Friday, though normally he was much earlier than this, often calling in for a quick drink after finishing work on his dress stall in the Northcote Road market.

'Hello, love. You're late today.'

'Yeah, Flo's gone to get us some fish and chips, so I thought I'd pop in.'

'You'd better make it a quick drink, then. You don't want Flo on your back.'

'Actually, Winnie, I'm not here for a drink. I've got something to tell you.'

Winnie felt her blood run cold. She could tell from Bill's face that what he had to tell her wasn't good. 'After last night, Bill, I knew there'd be bad news of some sort or other. Please, tell me, it isn't my Jan?'

'It's not Jan.'

'Thank Gawd for that. All right, don't beat about the bush.'

'It's Brian. I'm sorry, Winnie, but I've heard he's dead. He was killed last night.'

'Brian – my husband Brian?'

'Yes. I've been asking around all day but I don't know the details. A few of the blokes down the market have verified it though.'

Winnie wasn't sure how she should feel.

'Are you all right?'

'Yes. Yes, I'm fine, love. I suppose I should be crying but nothing's coming.'

'It's the shock. Where's Rachel?'

'She's upstairs.'

'I'll give her a shout,' Bill said. He went behind the bar and out to the back and then Winnie heard him calling for Rachel. She came down the stairs and Bill told her about Brian.

'I'll make you a cup of tea,' Rachel offered.

Winnie nodded but she'd rather have a glass of bubbly and celebrate. She felt terrible for feeling this way but it was the truth! Only she wasn't sure she should openly tell people that and decided it would be best to keep her feelings of joy to herself.

Once Rachel came back with a cup of tea, Bill said, 'I'd best get off. I'm sorry to be the bearer of such sad news, Winnie.'

'Thanks for coming to tell me, Bill. Make sure that you and Flo come in soon. There'll be a few drinks on the house waiting for you.'

'Thanks, Winnie. I'll be seeing you.'

'Are you sure you're all right?' Rachel asked quietly.

'Yes, love. More than all right. To tell you the truth, I'd sooner dance on his grave than waste any of my tears on him. But keep that to yourself; it's not becoming of a grieving widow. Blinkin' 'eck, I'm the merry widow! Shush though, don't let Lucy hear me talking about Brian like this.'

Shortly after Bill had left, Winnie stood with her cup in hand and quietly contemplated Brian's death. She'd be a lot better off now that she didn't have to share half the profits from the pub with him. But it wasn't the money that had left her feeling glad that Brian was gone. It was the feeling of freedom. It felt as though a huge weight had been lifted from her shoulders. That man could never bring her down or ever hurt her again.

18

On Saturday morning, after a restless night in the cellar, Lucy had spent a few hours in her bed tossing and turning. One minute, her mind was filled with dreamy images of marrying David; the next, she was almost overcome with fear at what she planned to do on Monday morning. But she'd do anything to make David happy and now, more than ever, he was going to need her support. She was dreading breaking the news to him of his father's death. Winnie hadn't seemed to be bothered and had hardly mentioned it. Once again, Lucy thought what a hard cow the woman was.

She heard a floorboard creak and checked the clock on her bedside table. It was early, but she was sure that Winnie was creeping down the stairs. Lucy was familiar with Winnie's routine and knew that the woman never ventured down to the pub until just before opening time. The last thing Lucy needed now was for Winnie to change her habits!

Lucy threw back the covers and wrapped her dressing gown around herself before quietly slipping from her room. She padded down the stairs and heard Winnie in the kitchen.

Just as she was about to turn on her heel and run back to her bedroom, Winnie saw her.

'Oh my Gawd, you frightened the bloomin' life out of me! What are you doing?' the woman asked.

'I thought I heard a noise. I was just checking. Sorry, I didn't mean to make you jump.'

'It's all right, love. Good on you for checking. The kettle's on, do want a cuppa?'

'No, thanks, I'm going to see if I can get another hour or two's sleep.'

'You're wide awake now; you may as well have a cup of tea.'

'Oh, go on, then,' Lucy answered with reluctance. She felt so guilty about her plans to rob Winnie, the last thing she really wanted to do was to sit at the kitchen table with her and share a pot of tea.

'It's nice and warm in the kitchen,' Winnie chirped, 'I've turned on all the gas rings.'

Lucy sat at the table and unconsciously chewed on her thumbnail. Her eyes fixed on the oven where she knew Friday's takings were hidden inside an old chocolate box. She'd always been stunned at Winnie's reluctance to use the safe upstairs but, as David had explained, his mother thought it was too obvious a place to steal from. Instead, Winnie had thought of the most unlikely location where a thief would look. *A thief.* Lucy was going to be a thief. She didn't like to associate the word with herself and quickly reasoned that it was only fair that David should have a cut of his mother's money.

'I couldn't sleep,' Winnie said and yawned. 'I thought it best to use the kitchen down here so that I didn't disturb anyone. Sorry for worrying you.'

'It's all right. I couldn't sleep either.'

'It's no wonder with bombs being dropped night after night. I should imagine you're like me, lying there awake and listening for the sound of planes and sirens.'

'Yes, I suppose I am.'

'It can't go on forever. Surely it's going to end soon. At this rate, there won't be much of London left. But let's not dwell on it, eh. There's plenty worse off than us. I mean, look at what happened to those poor buggers sheltering in Tottenham.'

'What happened?' Lucy asked.

'Didn't you hear? It was terrible, just terrible. A bomb landed right outside the shelter. Killed and injured loads.'

Lucy shuddered at the image conjured by Winnie's tale. It had only been a little while ago when she'd been running for her life as Battersea had taken the brunt of Hitler's force. She and David had escaped unscathed. They had been lucky that late afternoon. But the noise, the smells, the fear. The memories would be forever etched on her mind.

'There you go,' Winnie said as she placed a cup of tea on the table in front of Lucy. 'I can't start my day until I've had at least two cups.'

'Thank you,' Lucy replied, avoiding eye contact. 'I'm sorry about your husband.'

'Yeah, thanks, love. Don't worry about me, though. To tell you the truth, there was no love lost between me and him. I'm not grieving his death.'

Just then, Harry came into the kitchen. 'Good morning, ladies,' he greeted them. 'What are you doing down here?'

Lucy looked the man up and down, surprised to see that he was already dressed. Though she noticed that his dickie bow tie was a little crooked and his shirt was untucked on one side. She thought he must have dressed in a hurry.

'Oh, morning,' Winnie answered and she jumped up from her seat at the table and rushed to the sink. She threw her undrunk tea down the plughole and rinsed her cup and saucer.

'We came down here so that we wouldn't wake anyone,' Lucy answered Harry.

'I'm parched, is there any tea in the pot?' he asked.

'Yes, help yourself,' Winnie said shortly. 'I'm going upstairs to get dressed.'

'Actually, can I have a word please, Winnie?' Harry requested.

He looked at Lucy which prompted her to make her exit. 'Excuse me. I'll – erm – take this to my room,' she said. Lucy stood up and picked up her cup of tea, grateful to be away from Winnie. As she crept back up the stairs and looked at Rachel's closed bedroom door, her heart thudded. Stealing the money would be quite easy, as long as Winnie didn't wake too early. But tiptoeing into Rachel's room to take Martha would be far riskier. *A risk worth taking*, she thought, anything to make David love her.

Harry felt that Winnie seemed a bit off-hand with him. She'd been aloof all night in the cellar too. He knew it was nothing to do with Brian's death and had an inkling that Carmen had probably offended her.

'How are you this morning?' he asked, and offered her a wide smile.

'Fine, thanks. What did you want to talk to me about?' she answered abruptly.

Now there was no doubt in Harry's mind about Winnie's mood. 'Has my wife upset you?' he asked outright.

'No.'

'Have I?'

'No.'

'Only you seem a bit peeved with me.'

'Well, I'm not. I'm just tired, Harry.'

'Yeah, it's not been an easy few weeks. Is there anything I can do for you?'

'No, thank you.'

Harry wasn't convinced by Winnie's answer and wondered if they had outstayed their welcome. 'Me and Carmen are hoping to be moving out today. Carmen's on the lookout for something suitable. I hope you know how grateful we are to you.'

'No need for gratitude. We all have to help each other out at times like this.'

'There's every need, Winnie. You opened your home to us when no one else would have and you've been more than welcoming.'

Winnie was still standing at the sink and he thought he saw her bristle.

'I'm getting back on my feet,' he said, 'and once I'm straight, I'll see you're all right.'

'I've told you, there's no need. Your rations and the extras you've thrown in have been good enough.'

'But I'd like to treat you.'

Winnie sighed loudly and threw her dishcloth into the sink. 'I'd really rather you didn't,' she said sharply.

Harry walked across the small room towards her. 'Tell me what's bothering you, and don't say *nothing*. I'm no expert on women but I know when a lady has got the hump with me.'

'It's noth—' Winnie answered and she paused briefly before continuing. 'I mean, I'd rather not talk about it.'

'A problem shared. Are you more upset about Brian than you've been letting on?' he pushed.

'No, of course I'm not. The man was awful to me, you know all about him beating me. Look, just leave me be, Harry.'

'I can't do that. I don't like to see you like this. You know you can talk to me about anything. We're friends, aren't we?'

Winnie didn't answer and remained facing the sink.

'Well, aren't we?' he repeated, thinking about how he wanted so much more than just her friendship.

'Yes, we're friends. But your wife seems to think there's more to it!'

Ah, at last he'd got down to the crux of the problem. And as he'd suspected, Winnie's dark mood had been caused by Carmen. Christ, he wished his wife could have kept her mouth shut instead of spreading her poison and upsetting their kind and generous host. And he wished he could open up and tell Winnie that he loved her. But he couldn't and instead said, 'I don't know what Carmen has said to you but I'm sorry.'

'She hasn't said anything to me. I heard you both talking, yesterday, in the kitchen upstairs.'

'Ah, I see. Take no notice of what you heard, Winnie. It's just Carmen being Carmen. I'd hate for her to ruin our friendship.'

'Yeah, well, she has. We can't be friends, Harry, can't you see that?'

Harry was sure he heard Winnie sniff. 'Turn around and look at me,' he told her. His heart thudded. He couldn't lose her friendship.

Winnie shook her head. Harry drew closer to her and placed his hand on her shoulder. He could feel her trembling. Upset women normally made him uncomfortable but he felt the urge to wrap her in his arms and make her feel better. Of course, he didn't, but he wanted to.

'Are you crying?' he asked gently.

Winnie nodded.

'Please don't cry. I hate to see you this upset over my wife's wicked mind. Come on, Winnie, you're my best mate.' *And more*, he thought.

'I can't be your friend, Harry. You don't understand.'

Now he could hear that she was really sobbing.

'Come on, sweetheart, it's not as bad as all that,' he soothed.

'But it is, Harry; it's worse.'

'Tell me. Tell me what's wrong.'

'I can't,' she said through her tears.

Harry took hold of both her shoulders and tenderly turned her around to face him. She held her head down so he gently placed his finger under her chin and lifted her face. God, he wanted to kiss her so much.

'Now, out with it. I won't let you go until you tell me what's on your mind.'

Winnie drew in a juddering breath. 'I feel so stupid. I'm a foolish woman, Harry. Please, just leave me alone.'

'Not on your Nelly. I'm not leaving you in this state. What

sort of friend would that make me? Please, sweetheart, talk to me.'

'All right. I'll tell you. I love you,' Winnie blurted. 'There, now you know. Carmen was right and I'm a bloody idiot.'

Harry gazed at Winnie in astonishment, unsure at first if he'd heard her correctly. His mouth opened to speak but as he formed the words on his lips, Carmen's screeching voice interrupted.

'I knew it. I knew I was right all along about you two.'

Harry leapt back from Winnie. 'It's not what you think,' he said, knowing that his words sounded pathetic.

'It's exactly what I think. Carrying on under the same roof as me! How dare you treat me like this, you miserable excuse for a husband.' Then Carmen turned her attention to Winnie. 'And you, you fat tart! No wonder you was quick to offer us somewhere to stay. How convenient it must have been for you.'

'Don't talk to Winnie like that. There's nothing been going on with us. All she's done is been kind enough to house us.'

'You're defending her an' all!' Carmen screamed. 'It's bad enough that you've been sleeping with her but now you're sticking up for her over me!'

Rachel appeared behind Carmen. 'What's going on?' she asked, looking bewildered.

'Nothing, go back upstairs,' Winnie answered quickly.

'Nothing! Nothing! I'd hardly call it nothing!' Carmen shouted. 'Your landlady has been having an affair with my husband. Though God only knows what he sees in her. Jesus Christ, what sort of pub is this? You're all as bad as each other. Unmarried mothers, sluts and tarts. It's no bloody wonder that her husband left, God rest his soul, and now she's after mine!'

'That's enough!' Winnie yelled. 'Rachel, go back to your room. Carmen, pack your things and get out. For the record, I've not been having an affair with your husband and nor would I. But to be honest, how he hasn't run into the arms of another woman is beyond me. And if he did, no one would blame him. What's he got with you, eh? Just a cold, wicked, spiteful bitch. You don't deserve him.'

To Harry's horror but not his surprise, instead of turning around and marching off, Carmen flew across the room towards Winnie. Harry acted quickly and jumped in front of his wife. Her fingers came at his face. A sharp pain burned his skin as her nails ripped over his cheek, narrowly missing his eye. Harry tried to grab her wrists but Carmen was like a wildcat.

'I'll kill her, I swear, I'll bloody kill her,' Carmen hissed as she fought to get to Winnie.

'Calm down,' Harry said, grappling with her arms.

He managed to get a hold of one of her wrists but she slapped him hard across the face with her free hand. The whack stung and Harry was shocked at her strength and ferocity. He could hear Rachel in the background.

'Stop, please stop!' she cried.

Rachel's pleas did nothing to deter Carmen. His wife was kicking at his shins now.

'Get off me!' Carmen shrieked.

Harry caught her other flailing arm and gripped her tightly. 'Pack it in,' he growled.

Carmen instantly became still. But then she spat directly in his face.

'I hate you, Harry. But I'll *never* let *her* have you,' she said through gritted teeth.

Harry pulled his eyes away from Carmen's accusing glare. 'Can you leave us?' he said.

Winnie stepped out from behind him and slunk out of the kitchen with Rachel. Then he looked at his wife. 'If I let you go, will you promise to stay calm?'

Carmen gave him a filthy look but nodded in agreement.

When he released his grip on her, he braced himself but she didn't hit out at him. Instead, she spun around and headed for the stairs. Harry rushed after her, worried that Carmen was going to start a fight with Winnie.

'What are you doing?' he called as she stamped up the stairs.

'I'm leaving.'

'Where are you going?'

Carmen spun round at the top of the stairs and glared down at him. 'I don't know. But if you've got any respect for me, you'll pack your bags and leave with me.'

With that, she marched into the bedroom and slammed the door shut.

Harry, standing halfway up the staircase, stared at the closed bedroom door. Then his eyes fell on the kitchen door which was also shut. He knew that Winnie was behind that door, probably nursing her injured pride with a cup of tea and crying on Rachel's shoulder. His head told him to go after Carmen. But his heart wanted to be with Winnie. He trudged up the remaining stairs and stood on the landing in a dilemma. His life with Carmen would never be the same again. She'd hold this against him forever and make his life near unbearable. Whereas, almost within reach, there was a kind woman who loved him. Winnie was fun to be with and made him feel good. She offered the companionship that he'd never get from Carmen. Or from his *other* women.

The bedroom door opened and Carmen came out carrying a small bag. 'Well?' she asked sharply.

Harry glanced again at the kitchen door. He wanted to walk through it and sweep Winnie into his arms. But he didn't have the guts. Instead, with slumped shoulders and a heavy heart, he said, 'Just give me a minute to pack.'

As Harry threw his few belongings into a box, he knew he'd forever regret not following his heart. But as always, he'd taken the easy route and resigned himself to a loveless marriage with a spiteful woman who would never offer him the warmth and kindness that exuded from dear Winnie Berry.

19

The next morning, Winnie sat in the kitchen with Rachel and Hilda. She was pleased that Lucy was still in bed and hadn't pressed her about yesterday's events. After all, she hardly knew the girl. But Rachel and Hilda were like family to her and she was happy to open her heart to the women.

'I can't believe you told him how you feel,' Hilda said, shaking her head in disbelief.

'Me neither. It just came out. I felt such an idiot. Why, oh why couldn't I just keep me mouth shut!'

'And I can't believe he moved out with Carmen!' Rachel added.

'They're married, love. Carmen is his wife. He did the right thing. There was never any chance of me and Harry having any sort of future together. It was just a silly pipe dream on my part. I dunno, maybe this war is getting to me in strange ways.'

'Like I said, Win, you can't help who you fall in love with. But Rachel has made a good point. I'm surprised that Harry chose to stay with Carmen. She's an awful woman.'

'She's not all bad. No one is *all* bad. Everyone has redeeming features.'

'Yeah, like what? Name just one of Carmen's redeeming features,' Hilda challenged.

Winnie thought for a few moments. She struggled to think of anything positive to say about the woman. 'Carmen's got a good figure,' she finally said.

'And that's the best you can come up with?' Hilda asked.

'She's a good mum. She loves her kids and, let's be honest, Errol is a man that only a mother could love.'

'She's not a good mum,' Rachel argued. 'Cheryl has moved out and Errol – well, she raised a monster!'

'All right. She kept a good home and takes care of her appearance.'

'Face it, she's just a nasty woman and Harry is mad to put up with her,' Hilda said.

Winnie shook her head. 'She wasn't always such a hard bitch. I remember years back, when she first moved to Battersea. She was friendly and always smiling. I used to quite like her and so did everyone else.'

'We are talking about the same woman?' Rachel asked. 'Carmen?'

'Yes. It sounds silly now but I used to be a bit jealous of her. She was such a striking-looking woman and she was bubbly too. I was sure Brian used to fancy her.'

'Blimey, I can't imagine Carmen being *bubbly*,' Rachel said.

'I don't know what changed her over the years. I mean, it's not as if she's had a hard life. She's got a good husband and you can see he never kept her short. From what I can see, she's got nothing to be so bitter about.' Winnie sat in quiet contemplation as she watched Hilda pour her tea from her cup and into her saucer. She missed Harry. She used to look forward to having a cuppa with him in the mornings when Carmen was still sleeping. It would brighten her mood; she enjoyed starting the day with him. Oh, how she wished she hadn't blurted out her feelings. 'I'll probably never see him again,' she mumbled.

'I wouldn't bet on it,' Hilda said. 'He does good business in the pub. He'll be back.'

'I hope not! I don't think I could ever look him in the eye again.'

'Why? You've done nothing wrong.'

'I told a married man that I love him. That's wrong in my books.'

'I can't see Carmen allowing him to trade in here,' Rachel said.

'No, she'll never let him near me again,' Winnie said with a small chuckle. 'And she'll be telling everyone what a tart I am.'

'I wouldn't think so, Win, she hasn't got any friends to tell. But I reckon she'll be casting spells on you,' Hilda laughed.

'Blimey, I hope I don't turn into a frog. Ribbit, ribbit.'

They all chortled and Winnie began to feel better. She knew she'd always love Harry but he wasn't hers and never would be. But she had two beautiful women sitting around the table with her who would always be her friends. And Jan, her precious adopted daughter doing heroic and life-saving work at St Thomas's. She didn't need a man in her life to make her happy. She was already blessed and her life fulfilled. Harry was nothing more than a fanciful dream that was never going to come true.

★

'What's it like sleeping on the train platform underground?' Yvonne asked Cheryl.

'It's flamin' awful,' Edie answered.

'But at least we're safe down there,' Cheryl added. 'And now the Government have finally approved the use of the stations.'

'I forgot to tell you, Cheryl,' Yvonne said eagerly. 'Carol and Anne saw Lucy with Mrs Berry's son again. They said that she and David looked very lovey-dovey together.'

'Blimey! Has anyone told Mrs Berry?'

'I don't think so.'

'Perhaps you should mention it to her, Errol?' Cheryl suggested.

'It's nothing to do with me,' he answered.

'And I'm not getting involved either,' Yvonne said adamantly.

Cheryl huffed. 'Well, someone should tell her.'

'It's not Errol's or Yvonne's responsibility,' her gran added.

Cheryl felt awful that she couldn't let Mrs Berry know about Lucy and David. But if Errol and Yvonne were unwilling to tell the woman, then there was little that Cheryl could do about it.

Errol stuffed a biscuit into his mouth and swallowed it after just a few chews. 'These are lovely, Gran,' he said, reaching for another.

'Gran spent nearly all day baking yesterday,' Cheryl told them.

'I hope you didn't go to too much just trouble for us,' Errol said.

'It's not just for us.' Edie smiled.

They heard a knock on the door and Edie added, 'That'll be Bobby.'

Cheryl leapt to her feet. 'Oh, no, Gran, what have you done?'

'I invited him for tea and cake. I'm allowed to, you know, this is my house.'

'I know, Gran, but – but—'

'Stop flapping and go and let him in.'

'Who's Bobby?' Errol asked, frowning.

'He's a lovely lad who your sister is sweet on. So you make sure you're polite to him or I'll box your ears.'

There was a second knock and Cheryl's heart raced.

'Hurry up, you can't keep him waiting on the doorstep,' her gran said, shooing Cheryl with her hand.

Cheryl's mouth went dry. As she walked down the hallway, she straightened her dress and patted her hair. She couldn't believe her gran had orchestrated this. And to top it all, she'd be under her brother's scrutinising glare. *Poor Bobby*, she thought. He had no idea what he was about to walk into.

'Hello,' Cheryl greeted him, smiling broadly as she opened the door. 'You must be Bobby. My gran said she'd invited you.'

'Yes, hello. But I'm sorry, you seem to be at an advantage, as I don't know who you are.'

'I'm Cheryl. Cheryl Hampton. Edie's granddaughter. Please, come in.'

Cheryl pulled the door wider and stood back as Bobby walked through, his limp hardly evident. She leaned forward and whispered, 'I hope you won't feel like you're walking into an ambush. My best friend and older brother are in the front room with my gran.'

'Sounds like a party,' Bobby said, smiling.

Cheryl showed Bobby into the room and made brief introductions. The fact that Errol didn't smile or offer his hand to shake wasn't lost on Cheryl. She hoped it hadn't made Bobby feel uncomfortable but he seemed to be taking it all in his stride. Little did he know that his invite was a set-up and that Cheryl wanted to die of embarrassment.

'Bobby's a butcher, ain't that right?' Edie said. She then instructed Cheryl to pour him a cup of tea.

'Yes, that's right. I work in a shop on the High Road but hope to have my own one day.'

'Good for you, a man with ambition,' Edie said and she smiled. 'Our Cheryl works on the High Road too. She's in Barratt's shoe shop.'

'I could do with a new pair of boots,' Bobby said and he looked over at Cheryl.

She could feel her cheeks redden and noticed Errol's eyes boring into Bobby. 'Come in one day,' she said, 'I'm sure I could help you find a suitable pair.'

'What do you do, Yvonne?' Bobby asked.

'I work in a factory in Battersea.'

'And you?' he asked Errol.

'I mind me own business,' Errol answered with a scowl.

Cheryl cleared her throat and then asked lightly, 'Would you like another slice of cake?'

'It's delicious, thank you, but I haven't finished this piece yet.'

'Do you like it, Son?' Edie asked.

'Yes, it's very good cake.'

'Cheryl made it. She's ever such a good cook and keeps this place nice. She'd make someone a good wife.'

'Gran,' Cheryl hissed and she threw her gran a warning look.

But Edie continued and asked Bobby, 'Do you go out much? You know, to the local dances or anything.'

'No, not much. I've not had anyone to go with.'

'Oh, you should take Cheryl. She's only just moved over to Balham from Battersea. She doesn't know anyone around here. It would be nice for her to go out and not to have to be stuck here, cooped up with me.'

'Erm – yeah, sure,' Bobby answered and then he smiled at Cheryl.

If he hadn't noticed her blushes before, he must have done so now. Cheryl could feel herself glowing and wished her gran would stop being so obvious.

'Haven't you got any mates to go out with?' Errol quizzed Bobby.

'Yes, but most of them are busy with girls.'

'How come you ain't got a girl, then? What's wrong with you? You ain't one of them poofters are you?'

'There's nothing wrong with Bobby,' Edie snapped. 'He just hasn't found the right girl, ain't that right, dear?'

'Yeah, I suppose,' Bobby answered and he shifted uncomfortably in his seat.

'More tea?' Cheryl asked.

'Erm, no, thanks. I'd best be off. It's been nice meeting you all.'

'But you've only been here two minutes,' Edie moaned.

'Yes, sorry, I – erm – I forgot, I said I'd call in to see my gran. She'll be expecting me.'

'Cheryl, see the man out.'

Bobby stepped out of the front door and then turned to Cheryl. 'It really was nice to meet you,' he said.

'Yes, you too. I'm sorry about them.'

'Don't worry, your brother was just being a good brother and looking out for his sister. But what your gran said about going out — would you like that?'

'Yes, I would.'

'Right, then, I'll pick you up next Sunday at one. Is that all right?'

'Yes, that's great. I'll see you next week.'

Cheryl closed the door and leaned against it for a moment to gather her thoughts. She couldn't believe that her gran and Errol hadn't put Bobby off. She stormed back into the front room. 'How could you? What on earth must Bobby have thought?'

'Did he ask you out?' her gran asked.

'Yes.'

'So stop complaining.'

'And you, Errol, you were so rude!'

'Like Gran said, stop complaining.'

'Oh, so you've no objections to me going out with him?'

'No, he seems nice enough,' Errol answered and he winked at their gran.

Cheryl looked at Yvonne but her friend was peering doe-eyed at Errol. 'Maybe Bobby will have a friend that you could go out with. We could double date,' Cheryl suggested.

'I'm not sure about that,' Yvonne answered awkwardly.

'I am. I'll pop into the butcher's in the week and ask him. If he has, Errol can bring you over to stay with us next Saturday. Though we'll probably end up down the tube station.'

'I'm not a taxicab service,' Errol said.

'Don't worry, dear, I'll make some more of them biscuits for you,' Edie said, smiling.

Errol didn't protest and Cheryl could see that he was quite taken with their gran. And so he should be. Edie had a way about her that made you feel warm and cosy, nothing like their mother, who would have you walking on eggshells around her. Cheryl wished her gran had been in her life. They'd missed out on so many years. She stood up and walked over to Edie, then bent down and kissed the old lady on the cheek. 'Thanks,' she said.

'What for?'

'For being you.'

The gesture seemed to touch her gran. Edie pulled a handkerchief from the sleeve of her cardigan and dabbed her eyes. 'I'm so happy to have my grandchildren in my life,' she sniffed.

Cheryl and Errol exchanged a glance and, in that moment, Cheryl knew that her brother felt the same as she did. They both detested their parents for the lies and deceit. But most of all, they hated them for keeping them away from their grandmother.

A couple of hours later, Cheryl saw Errol and Yvonne to the front door.

'I'll see you on Saturday,' Errol said.

'Yes, and thanks for bringing Yvonne over.'

'Anytime. It gives me a good excuse to see the old girl. She's a character.'

'She is indeed. I think the world of her.'

'Yeah, me an' all,' Errol said warmly. But then his face darkened and the tone of his voice deepened. 'I'll never forgive my mother and Harry for what they've done. And I reckon that Harry deserves to learn a lesson.'

Errol went to walk away but alarm bells rang in Cheryl's head and she grabbed his arm. 'Wait, what do you mean?' she asked.

'Gran should never have been left alone and we shouldn't have been kept in the dark. I'm going to make sure that Harry pays for this.'

'How? What are you going to do?'

'Never you mind.'

'You can't beat him up, Errol. He's still my father, whether you like it or not.'

'Give me some credit, Sis. I'm not going to beat him up. But I am going to make sure that he realises what a bastard he's been. See ya.'

Cheryl watched Errol drive off with Yvonne, her stomach in knots. Errol had never been one for making idle threats but at least he'd agreed not to beat her dad up. She dreaded to think what her brother had in store for him. And though she'd never wish any harm to come to her parents, she hoped that Errol would make their mother pay too.

She tried to dismiss the thoughts from her head. She had the date with Bobby to look forward to but now that Errol had said what he'd said, a dark cloud hung over her, over-shadowing everything.

20

On Monday morning, Lucy lay in bed feeling sick. She hadn't even bothered trying to get any sleep. The minutes ticked by slowly, each one that passed bringing her closer to the moment that would change her life forever. She sat up and pulled the covers over her knees whilst staring at her bedroom door. Once again, she ran through a mental check list. Everything was in place. She just needed to summon the courage to go through with it.

Tick. Tick. Tick. Lucy tried to listen to the sound of the clock instead of the noise of her heart thumping in her ears. *Tick. Tick. Tick.* The time was getting closer.

Trying to be as quiet as she could, Lucy threw her legs over the edge of her bed and slipped her feet into her slippers. She pulled her dressing gown around herself to hide the fact that she was fully dressed. Then, tiptoeing to the door, she held her ear against it and listened. The place was in silence. Rachel and Martha were asleep in the room next door and Winnie was in her own bed again, further along the passage-way. Thank goodness Mr and Mrs Hampton had moved out. That was two less people to worry about.

Lucy squinted in the dark to look at the clock again. It was time. She had to act now before anyone woke and captured her in the act of stealing the pub's takings and snatching Martha. Doubts crept into her mind and she tried to push them away. *You're doing this for David. For you to be a proper family*, she reminded herself.

As she bent down to pull her packed bag from under the bed, she heard a small whimper from Martha next door. Lucy froze and held her breath. She squeezed her eyes closed. *Please don't wake up Rachel*, she thought, her jaw tense and her stomach churning. Thankfully, Martha quietened.

Then, as quiet as a mouse, Lucy opened the door. She popped her head through and looked along the dark passageway before sneaking out and down the stairs.

Damn it! She'd forgotten about the creaky floorboard and she paused, praying that Winnie and Rachel hadn't heard it. When their doors didn't open, she carried on down. Relief flooded through her as she walked into the kitchen. She'd done it. But she was far from in the clear yet.

Feeling giddy with nerves, Lucy opened the oven and grabbed the chocolate box. Her pulse raced and sweat began to form on her brow. Quickly stuffing the box of money into her bag, she rushed to the back door and shoved the bag under a blanket in Martha's pram.

It would have been so easy to run through the back door now and get clean away with David but she knew he'd be disappointed if she didn't show up with Martha.

Lucy crept back up the stairs again, this time remembering to step over the creaky floorboard. She stood outside Rachel's bedroom and reached for the door handle. Her hand was trembling visibly. She drew in a breath, trying to calm herself. *You can do this*, she said in her head. She was so close now.

Slowly pushing the door open, Lucy crept into the room. She could see Rachel's head resting on the pillow, the covers pulled up under her chin. Martha's cot sat at the end of the bed. One, two, three, four, five light steps and now she was leaning over the cot and reaching down to scoop up Martha. The baby stirred and whined. Lucy pulled her into her chest to muffle the noise. She glanced at Rachel who remained asleep.

One, two, three, four, five steps and she was almost out of the door. She heard a noise from behind and stood motionless. Rachel was moving. *Please don't wake up.* But Lucy was prepared. She had her story ready. She'd say that she heard Martha crying and had come in to see to her so that Rachel could sleep. Would Rachel believe her? Lucy hoped she wouldn't have to put her story to the test. She glanced over her shoulder, still holding Martha tightly to her chest. Rachel had turned over in the bed and was now facing the wall.

Lucy didn't hesitate any longer and dashed out of the door, leaving it ajar before fleeing down the stairs. As she pulled Martha from the closeness of her chest, the baby howled. Lucy, panicking, held her hand over Martha's tiny face. 'Please be quiet, little one,' she whispered.

Martha's cries couldn't be heard but Lucy knew that as soon as she removed her hand, the baby would scream. She fiddled with the back door, trying to open it with a baby in her arms and a hand over the baby's mouth. What felt like an eternity only took a few moments and the door was open. She dashed through it, pushing the pram and holding the baby.

She ran as fast as she could until she was at the end of the street and around the corner. Here, she stopped briefly to put the crying child into the pram and swapped her slippers for her shoes. She stuffed them and her dressing gown into the pram and then continued to run.

After a while, as Lucy came closer to Clapham Junction railway station, Martha finally stopped crying, the motion of the pram sending her back to sleep.

The sun hadn't yet risen but she could see a lone figure waiting outside the station. She was early but she hoped it was David. She wouldn't feel safe until she was on the train with him and far away from Battersea. She'd wait until they were in Richmond before she'd break the tragic news to him about his father's death.

'David, thank goodness you're here,' Lucy gushed breathlessly. 'I did it.'

'I knew you wouldn't let me down,' he said, pulling her into his arms. 'The pram was a good idea to hide your bag.'

'And to carry Martha,' Lucy said. 'I couldn't have managed without it.'

'What do you mean, *to carry Martha*?'

'I couldn't have lugged her and my bag all the way here without the pram.'

David pulled away from her and leaned over the pram. He pulled the cover back and gaped at the sleeping child. 'Where's the money?' he asked.

'In my bag,' Lucy answered proudly.

David opened the bag and grabbed the box. He took the money out and shoved it into his pockets before throwing the box back into the pram. 'You stupid cow,' he said scathingly. 'Why did you bring her?' he asked, pointing at Martha.

'I-I-I thought that was what you wanted – I thought you wanted us to be a family.'

'When did I ever suggest to you that you should steal Martha from Rachel, eh?'

'I-I don't know. You wanted me to take her, I know you did, David.'

'No, Lucy, I didn't. If I take that child, Rachel, my mother and just about every copper in London will be looking for me. Do you think Rachel will ever stop looking? My God, are you thick?'

Tears began to prick at Lucy's eyes. This wasn't how she'd expected David to react. 'I thought—'

'You didn't think, though, did you? If you had done, you'd never have brought *that* with you!'

Martha began to wake so Lucy tucked the blankets back over her. 'We've got her now. I can't take her back and we can't leave her here. She'll have to come with us but think about it, David, it'll be perfect. You, me and Martha, a proper family.'

'You're off your rocker. I don't want to be lumbered with her or to spend the rest of my life looking over my shoulder.'

Lucy stood numb with shock as David turned to walk away. 'Wait,' she called, 'what are we going to do?'

David spun back around and stamped angrily towards her. His face was so close to hers that she could feel his spittle on her cheek. '*We* ain't going to do anything. I'm going. This is your mess; you can sort it.'

'But what about me?' Lucy cried as he walked away. She left the pram and ran after him, grabbing at his arm. 'Please, David, wait. You can't leave without me.'

David shook her off and spoke with venom. 'I never

wanted you in the first place. I know all about you, how you've always been desperate for a husband and about how you falsely accused a bloke of attacking you. You're a nutter. I played you, Lucy, and you was happy to do my bidding. Now, piss off.'

Lucy, shocked and bereft, watched through her tears as David strode into the train station. As he disappeared from sight, she peeked over her shoulder at the pram and heard Martha crying. What was she going to do? She couldn't return to the pub. What if they had discovered that the money and the baby were gone?

Her legs felt weak but she managed to run after David. The lights from inside the station felt bright. She blinked hard and then she saw him turn a corner and head for a platform. Lucy gave chase. 'David – David!' she called. 'Wait – please, wait for me.' But David marched on.

When she caught up with him on the platform, he looked at her angrily. 'I told you to piss off,' he growled.

'I love you. Please, we can make this work.'

David shook his head. 'I'm not interested, Lucy. I've got the money, that's all I wanted. Now, do us both a favour and leave me alone.'

'I don't believe you. You love me, you told me you wanted me to be your wife. You said that you would marry me. Please, give me a chance and I promise I'll make you happy,' she begged desperately and then she threw herself at his feet.

'Get up,' David barked. 'You're making a fool of yourself. I can't make it any clearer, Lucy. I don't want you and I never have.'

Lucy heard the rumbling sound of a train approaching the platform. She sat in a heap on the ground and gazed after

David as he walked away to board the incoming train. She'd lost him. No amount of crying or pleading would ever bring him back. David was about to get on a train and she knew she'd never see him again. She'd been left with nothing and only trouble to look forward to.

Slowly, Lucy pushed herself to her feet. The train was approaching fast. She walked to the edge of the platform, teetering dangerously close to the edge. Steam billowed out behind the train and the brakes began to screech.

'David!' she shouted. 'Goodbye.'

As Lucy stepped off the platform and into the path of the incoming locomotive, she saw David turn to look at her, his eyes wide as he screamed, 'Noooo!'

Then there was a thud. And she was gone forever.

21

Winnie quietly pulled Rachel's bedroom closed and trudged through to the kitchen. It felt strangely empty without Harry pouring her a fresh cuppa. She put the kettle on the stove and then reached for the biscuit tin. Now that Brian and David were no longer here, she kept her best biscuits upstairs instead of in the tin downstairs. Huh, Brian – dead. It was still sinking in. She'd dreamed about him in the night and her dreams had evoked some of the very few good memories she had of the man. She'd spent most of their lives together in fear of him. Winnie bristled. She wouldn't allow any sadness over his death to creep in. He wasn't worth her tears. She'd cried enough of them when they'd been together. Instead, she thought of Harry again. She was free to be with whoever she wanted but the fact remained that Harry was still very much a married man. And even if he wasn't, Winnie didn't believe that he'd ever think of her as anything other than a friend. *Good grief*, she thought, chastising herself for still wanting him.

'Where's my girl?' Rachel asked and yawned. 'Thanks for seeing to her, Win. I didn't hear her wake up.'

Winnie turned around confused and looked at Rachel. 'What do you mean, love?'

'Martha. I must have slept through her crying. Did she wake you?'

'No, I've not heard her.'

'You didn't take her from her cot this morning?'

'No.'

Rachel's eyes stretched wide. 'Where is she, then?' she asked, the panic in her voice evident.

'I don't know, love. She must be in with Lucy.'

Both women rushed from the kitchen and along the passageway. Rachel rapped on Lucy's bedroom door. When there was no answer, Winnie urgently instructed, 'Open it.'

They stood there aghast, peering at the empty room.

'She's taken Martha! Oh my God, Winnie, she's stolen my baby!'

'Calm down, she's probably just gone out for a walk with her,' Winnie soothed, trying to sound relaxed. Though in reality, her words felt empty and her stomach was twisting.

'Out for a walk at this time of the morning? I doubt it,' Rachel cried. She marched into Lucy's room and opened the drawers. 'Her clothes have gone.'

Winnie gulped. It was quickly becoming clear what had happened here. Intuitively, she knew that Lucy had run off with Martha and David was behind it. 'Try not to worry. We'll get her back. I'm going to throw some clothes on and then I'll go to the phone box and call the police.'

Rachel nodded and then pushed past Winnie and headed for the stairs.

'Where are you going?' Winnie called.

'To find my baby!'

'But you're not dressed.'

Rachel was at the bottom of the stairs now and didn't reply.

'Rachel—'

Winnie heard the back door close. She stood in her empty flat feeling helpless, her heart racing. Then she remembered. The police. She had to call the police. Spurred into action, she dashed to her bedroom, threw on her clothes and then hurried to the telephone box.

She bumped into Len, coming from the shop with his morning newspaper. 'Lucy has run off with Martha. Have you seen her?'

'No, but I'll spread the word. Have you called the police?'

'On my way now. I can't stop, Len. Get everyone you can round to the pub. I need as many people as possible to go out looking for them.'

'Will do. I'll knock 'em up, if I have to. Go, call the police.'

After a frantic telephone call, the police told Winnie that they would send someone straight to the pub. When Winnie returned, she was grateful to see that Len had managed to gather at least a dozen men.

'There's more coming,' he told Winnie.

She dashed around to the back door to let herself in. 'Rachel! Rachel!'

There was no answer. The poor, frantic girl must still be running around Battersea in her nightclothes.

Winnie opened the pub doors. 'Thank you very much,' she said, tears welling in her eyes. 'It appears that Lucy has run off with my granddaughter, probably with David. Please, search everywhere you can think of. I need my granddaughter back home.'

'Don't worry, Winnie. If they're in Battersea, one of us will find them.'

Winnie, overcome with emotion and unable to speak now, nodded.

The men filed out of the pub. Winnie steadied herself by holding on to the edge of the bar. The door burst open again and Hilda flew in.

'Is it true? Has Lucy kidnapped Martha?'

'Yes, love.'

'Oh, Winnie, what are we going to do? Where's Rachel?'

'She's out looking for her, and so are a load of my customers. I've called the police; they're on their way here.' Winnie tried to stop the tears from falling. She wanted to be strong for Rachel. But she couldn't and a sob caught in her throat.

'Pack that in, Win. It's not the time for tears. Our beautiful granddaughter will be home soon, you'll see.'

'Yes, you're right.' Winnie sniffed. 'I think it's just the shock.'

'Sit down, I'll make us a cuppa.'

As Winnie went to take a seat, another thought struck her. 'I bet Lucy has robbed me of my money an' all,' she said solemnly.

Hilda followed Winnie into the kitchen. Winnie opened the oven and her heart sank again. 'It's gone,' she said. 'But, to be honest, I don't care about the money. I just want Martha home.'

They heard a male voice call through from the bar.

'That'll be the police,' Hilda said.

Winnie hurried back into the pub.

'Mrs Berry?' the constable asked.

'Yes, thank you for coming so quickly. As I explained on the telephone, Lucy Little, my barmaid and lodger, has run off with my granddaughter, Martha Berry. She's only a baby. You must find her.'

'Yes, yes, Mrs Berry, we've already got men out looking for them. I've several questions for you. Perhaps we can sit down?'

'I'll fetch tea,' Hilda said.

Winnie pulled out a seat at a table but couldn't sit still. Her legs jigged nervously and her hands shook.

'Do you have any idea where Miss Little would have taken the baby?'

'No. Well, yes, to my son, I suppose, but I don't know where he is.'

'Your son?'

'Yes, David Berry. He's the baby's father but he ran off months ago.'

'And where is the baby's mother?'

'Running around Battersea in her nightclothes looking for Martha.'

'I see. And why do you think that Miss Little took the child?'

'I don't know; she's mad. She's pinched the weekend's takings too. Look, I don't mean to be rude, but this is wasting time. You should be out there looking for my granddaughter!'

'As I explained, there are already officers looking.'

Winnie hung her head. 'I'm sorry. I'm just frantic with worry. What if they've got on a train somewhere and have left Battersea? Will we ever find them?'

'Please, try to stay calm.'

The door burst open again and more of Winnie's customers came in. Hilda quickly explained the situation to them and the men rushed off. Everyone could sense the need for urgency. So many people had joined the search. Surely they'd find dear Martha?

Harry had been awake for a while and he was sitting quietly, looking through the bedroom window. They'd rented a double room in a house, just for now until they could find something more suitable. This place was far from ideal. Carmen had already said that she hated sharing a house and she had threatened Harry, saying that he'd better pull his finger out. But she'd refused to spend another night under Winnie's roof so, reluctantly, they had accepted this room in desperation.

He peered more closely through the window. There seemed to be a bit of a commotion going on outside. He was shocked to see Rachel in her nightclothes. The girl looked frantic. He wondered what the hell was going on. Had something terrible happened to Winnie?

Harry, with his heart racing, quickly and quietly pulled on his clothes before running down the stairs and out onto the street. A small group of people had gathered around Rachel.

'What's going on?' he asked urgently.

'Harry – have you seen Lucy? She's stolen my baby!'

Harry sighed with relief, pleased that Winnie was fine and safe. 'No, sweetheart, I've not seen her. Have you called the police?'

'Yes, Winnie was going to do that.'

He placed his arm over her shoulder. Her body was trembling, possibly because it was quite nippy out but more likely it was due to shock. 'Come on, I'm taking you home. You can't run around the streets in your nighty. The police will find your baby.'

'No, Harry, no! I can't go home, not without Martha.'

'She might already be at home. You'll catch your death out here,' he said and urged her along the street. He took his coat off and draped it over her shoulders. Cor, there really was a biting nip in the air. The poor girl must be cold down to her bones, he thought.

Rachel cried and mumbled for most of the walk. But as they turned the corner, she suddenly sprinted off towards the pub. Harry tried to keep up with her but he couldn't. When, finally, he got to the Battersea Tavern, Rachel was already inside and he was breathless. It was at times like this that Harry really felt his age.

He pushed the door open to see Rachel sobbing in Winnie's arms.

'I see she's got your coat. Thanks for bringing her back,' Hilda whispered.

'What's going on? I couldn't get much sense out of her.'

'Lucy has kidnapped Martha and pinched Winnie's takings. We reckon she's gone off with David. There's loads of people looking for them. But so far, nothing.'

'Christ, that's terrible.'

'I know. We're all beside ourselves. I feel so useless, Harry. I wish that there was something I could do.'

'Just be there for Rachel. She'll need you and Winnie more than ever right now.'

'Yes, I know. I'll make more tea. That's all I seem to be good for at the moment. Tea, tea and more bloody tea.'

Hilda left quietly but not before Harry had seen the unshed tears in her eyes. This was a tragic situation and Harry felt that he was intruding. He was just about to turn around and sneak back out of the pub when Winnie caught his eye. Gawd, his heart broke for her. She looked so forlorn.

'Have you seen or heard anything?' she asked as she walked towards him.

'No, sweetheart, sorry. I saw Rachel in the street in a right state so I brought her home. The poor girl, she was frantic.'

'I know, we all are. I can't think where Lucy could be. I'm worried sick that she's jumped on a train to somewhere. It seems obvious to me. I mean, she ain't likely to stay around here knowing that everyone will be searching for her.'

Harry was about to offer some reassurance but the door opened and two policemen walked in. From the expressions on their faces, Harry thought they must have some awful news. Winnie must have thought so too because she gasped and grabbed hold of Harry's hand.

Rachel came running over and so did Hilda. Harry didn't feel that he should be there but with Winnie gripping his hand, he couldn't slip away.

'Have you found her? Have you found my baby?' Rachel asked, her eyes desperately searching the policemen's faces for a clue.

'Yes, Miss Robb. At least, we have found *a* baby that we believe to be Martha. She's safe and well and has been taken to hospital, just to be checked over. If you'd – erm – like to get dressed, we will take you to her.'

Rachel's legs must have given way. She slumped to the floor, crying in a heap. Winnie let go of Harry's hand and helped Hilda to get Rachel back on her feet.

'Take her upstairs to dress,' Winnie whispered to Hilda.

Once out of sight, Winnie asked the constable, 'Where did you find Martha?'

'At Clapham Junction railway station.'

'I knew it! I knew that cow would be trying to get on a train away from here. I hope you've arrested the pair of them, Lucy and my son.'

'I'm sorry, Mrs Berry, but we've some unfortunate news.'

'What? The baby is all right, isn't she?'

'Yes. But we couldn't find your son and Lucy Little – she threw herself under a train. We're sorry to inform you that she's dead. Her mother has been asked to formally identify her but it's just a formality. We know it's Miss Little and there's no reason to suspect foul play.'

'She had Martha!'

'Yes, the child was found in her pram outside the station.'

Winnie swayed and Harry thought that Winnie's legs were about to give way too. He quickly placed an arm around her waist.

'It's fine. I'm fine, thanks, Harry. It's just the thought of Lucy under a train and she could have taken Martha with her. Thank Gawd she didn't. Best not to mention any of this to Rachel at the moment.'

Rachel and Hilda came down the stairs. 'Take me to my baby,' Rachel demanded.

'I'll go with her. Do you want to come an' all, Win?' Hilda asked as she handed Harry his coat.

'No, love. You two go. I'll see you when you get back.'

Once they'd left, Winnie said, 'I need to get the search called off. There's loads of folk out looking.'

'Leave it to me,' Harry offered.

'Thanks, you've been ever so good.'

'Let's have a quick cuppa first, eh? You're shaking, Winnie, I don't want to leave you like this.'

'No, really, Harry, I'm fine. I just can't believe what's happened … Lucy, dead. David's to blame for this, I swear he is. It's awful to say but I wish I'd never given birth to that boy.'

Harry was thoughtful for a moment. He'd never regret

having Cheryl but he'd been left with a bitter taste in his mouth when it came to Errol. And the irony was, Errol wasn't even his son.

Harry led Winnie to a table. 'I'll fetch the tea. I know my way around,' he said with an uncomfortable small chuckle.

When he returned, he saw that Len was just leaving.

'Len popped in. There's no need to call off the search. Len will see to it. Thanks, though, Harry.'

'Good. That means I don't have to rush off and can sit with you.' Their eyes locked and, once again, Harry felt the urge to throw his arms around her.

'I was warned about Lucy,' Winnie said, breaking the awkward moment. 'Your Cheryl and her friends warned me. But I'd never have expected this.'

'Yeah, I'd heard rumours about her too but she seemed like a nice enough girl.'

'Her poor mother, having to go and identify her. She'll never get the image of her daughter's mangled body out of her head. It doesn't bear thinking about.'

'They won't show her mother, not if it's a mess.'

'Gawd, Harry, ain't it terrible. Don't get me wrong, I was ready to skin the girl alive but to throw herself under a train like that. She was so young. What on earth must have been going through her mind?'

'I wouldn't like to think, Winnie.'

'I reckon my David must have got her to do his dirty work and then he left her. Just like he did Rachel. But why did he run off without Martha? It doesn't make any sense. I don't suppose we'll ever know the truth. Not unless the police catch up with him and that's unlikely.'

The door opened again. Harry looked over his shoulder, horrified to see that Carmen was steaming towards the table.

'I should have known I'd find you in here with *her*!' she snarled.

Harry jumped to his feet. 'Carmen, just slow down, sweetheart. A terrible thing happened this morning.'

'I know. I've heard about that bastard child being kidnapped and about Lucy killing herself. That's how I knew you'd be in here. You can't help yourself, can you? You have to play the hero. Good old Harry, running to the rescue to sort everything out. Well, it's a shame you don't do the same for your wife!'

Winnie, looking too exhausted to rise to her feet, stated calmly, 'Just get out, Carmen. This is my pub and you and your spiteful tongue ain't welcome in here.'

'Don't worry, I'm going. And so is my husband. You can take a good, long look at him as he walks out because, believe you me, it'll be the last time you'll ever see him.' Carmen then turned to Harry and snapped, 'Come on, out.'

Harry breathed in deeply. He was tempted to tell Carmen to bugger off. But if he dared to stand up to her, she'd likely make even more of a scene. His wife had already belittled him and he dreaded to think what else she'd pull from her sleeve to make him feel small. And there were things that Carmen could say about him that he hoped would never reach Winnie's ears.

Harry looked at Winnie and mouthed, 'Sorry,' before trudging after his wife. As he followed in Carmen's wake, he began to ask himself what sort of a man he had become, to be ruled and shamed by his wife? It was like being married to his mother. Edie had always undermined him and had made him feel like second fiddle to her precious Wilf. Harry had been so jealous of Wilf. He'd felt he'd got one up on his brother when he'd stolen Carmen from him. But now Harry felt he'd lost his voice and wasn't himself around the woman and he wished he'd never taken her away from his brother. But with Winnie, it was different. She made him feel like a real bloke: Needed and wanted. And he could have a laugh and a joke with her. Harry was at last honest with himself. He wanted to be with Winnie and not Carmen. And Winnie, now widowed, had declared her love for him. The only obstacle that stopped them from being together was Carmen. He'd have to find the courage to tell his wife that he was leaving her. He'd get her settled in a house first and then break the news. Finding her a decent home was the least he could do. Carmen would get over it. Her pride would be hurt, especially when she discovered that he'd gone off to be with another woman. And to make it worse, that woman would be Winnie Berry.

22

It had been four days since Lucy had kidnapped Martha and Rachel hadn't allowed the baby out of her sight. Not that Winnie could blame the girl. It had been a terrifying experience for all of them but especially for Rachel.

Winnie wished that she'd taken more notice of what Carol and Cheryl had said about Lucy. But she hadn't, instead preferring to give Lucy a chance to prove herself. Winnie wouldn't make that mistake again. In future, though it went against the grain for her, she'd take more notice of rumours and gossip. After all, there was rarely any smoke without fire. And since Lucy's untimely demise, more gossip about her unsavoury character had spread through the borough. She'd never wish the girl dead, of course not, but she wasn't upset to see the back of her. And David too. Winnie refused to waste any more tears on her son. She hoped that she'd seen the last of him for good and that the police would eventually catch up with him. David deserved to be severely punished for his role in Martha's kidnap and Lucy's death, though Winnie suspected that no one would ever know the truth about what really happened on that station platform.

Len interrupted her thoughts. Sitting on his usual stool at the end of the bar, he asked for another bottle of stout.

Winnie placed the bottle on the counter in front of him and picked up his empty one. 'There you go, love. Sorry, I was miles away.'

'Best place to be,' Len replied.

'Cor, yeah, I wish we could be, Len. Mind you, it ain't just London that's being bombed. I don't think there's any big towns or cities that are safe from Hitler's planes.'

'Our boys are doing their best. The newspaper this morning said that about twenty Nazi machines were shot down over the Bristol Channel and Kent. Yet the slippery gits still get past. They were flying low last night. I could hear they had full loads an' all.'

'We can't hear much down in the cellar, which is a blessing, I suppose. Sometimes it's better not knowing what's coming, if you know what I mean,' Winnie said quietly, and she glanced over at Rachel and Martha, her heart full of concern.

'I know what you mean, Winnie,' Len answered gravely.

Every night, when the German planes came and unloaded their bombs on London, no one knew if they were going to wake up the next morning or if they'd be blown to smithereens in their sleep. Winnie had seen and heard such appalling things. Things she'd sooner forget but which she knew she never would. She didn't know how Jan coped at the hospital, all credit to the girl for having a strong stomach. And there was no doubt about it, a strong stomach was required when it came to dealing with folk who'd been caught up in an explosion. That's what Winnie had meant when she'd said to Len that it was better not to know what was coming. She'd prefer to be killed instantly rather than be left with agonising burns or parts of her body blown off. And she'd prefer not to know that death was coming. She wondered if Brian had known. As much as she had disliked her husband, she hoped he hadn't died in pain.

When the door opened and Winnie saw Errol saunter in, her jaw clenched. She hoped he'd behave himself without Harry around to keep him in line.

Errol moseyed up to the bar. 'Have you seen Harry?' he asked.

'No, he ain't been in all week. Not since Monday.'

'Do you know where he is?'

'Not a clue. Your mum and dad moved out at the weekend; I've no idea where to. But I'm sure if you ask around, someone's bound to know where your dad is.'

'He ain't my dad,' Errol said, snarling.

Winnie was taken aback. She'd known there'd been some family discord within the Hamptons. Harry had raised his doubts about Errol being his, but she hadn't realised that Errol knew too.

'I'll have half a pint while I'm here.'

Winnie tried to throw him a friendly smile but she'd rather Errol left without a drink. Nevertheless, she went ahead and poured him one.

'Sorry to hear about what happened with Rachel's kid and Lucy. Taking a baby like that, it ain't on. I heard David had something to do with it?'

'Yep, apparently so.'

'He's always been a wrong 'un.'

'You can say that again,' Winnie said.

'You deserve better, Mrs Berry.'

'Thank you, and yeah, I do,' Winnie chuckled. She was

surprised to find herself having a reasonable conversation with Errol.

'All that stuff a while back with David owing me money. I shouldn't have involved you. I hope I didn't upset you.'

'Actually, you did. But I'm willing to let bygones be bygones, just so long as you watch yourself in here.'

'You have my word, Mrs Berry. 'Ere, for you,' Errol said and he pulled a bar of chocolate from his coat pocket.

'It's all right; I don't need a gift from you.'

'I want you to have it. And there'll be plenty more gifts coming your way.'

'Oh yeah, why's that?'

'I'm going to be selling from here, if that's all right with you?'

'Selling what?' Winnie asked.

'Anything you like, Mrs Berry. I'm open for business and taking orders,' Errol answered.

He beamed widely and his eyes twinkled just like Harry's. For the first time, Winnie saw a bit of Errol's charm, a chip off the old block. 'I see. So you're helping your father out and following in his footsteps. Well, me and Harry have a good arrangement so I don't see any reason why it shouldn't work with you too.'

'Thanks, Mrs Berry. I'll see you're well looked after. And please stop calling Harry my *father*.'

'Whatever you say. But I'm warning you. The first sniff of trouble from you, or if you try and intimidate any of my customers, I'll sling you out of 'ere faster than a fart out of a dog with the trots.'

Errol smiled again. 'You won't get any trouble from me.' He finished his drink and wiped the back of his hand across his mouth. 'If you see Harry, tell him I'm looking for him. I'll be seeing you very soon.'

Rachel, with Martha in her arms, came to stand beside Winnie.

'What was all that about?' she asked.

'I don't know, love, but he's calling his father Harry and saying that Harry ain't his dad. Gawd knows what's gone on. Harry mentioned something about it too, but keep it to yourself. Anyway, they can't have fallen out too badly as Errol is on about flogging his gear in here, just like Harry does.'

'Is he going into business with Harry or setting up in competition?'

'I don't know. Oh, bugger, I just assumed he was working with Harry and I've given him the go ahead. What if he's working against him? I don't want trouble in here with the pair of them.'

'He wouldn't go against Harry – would he?'

'I wouldn't put anything past Errol.'

'At least he sounded like he was being polite to you.'

'He was. Maybe he's grown up, Rachel. Perhaps he ain't a thug no more. Or maybe David brings out the worse in people.'

'Hmm, maybe. But Errol still has a name for himself all over Battersea. I wouldn't trust him as far as I could throw him. I'm taking Martha up for a feed. Will you be all right down here by yourself?'

'Yes, love, its quiet enough,' Winnie answered with a smile. Though she supposed she should probably be thinking about hiring another person to work behind the bar. Only, this time, she'd be more careful about who she allowed to live under her roof with her most precious treasure – her darling granddaughter, Martha.

★

'There's not much to unpack. I'm off out for a pint,' Harry told Carmen.

In their new house, she'd been busy giving the cooker a once over but she spun around quickly. 'You'd better not be thinking about going to the Battersea Tavern.'

'No, I'll be in the Halfway House. I need to make some money to pay for this place.'

Thankfully, Carmen went back to examining her new kitchen and didn't question him further. But Harry felt sure that his wife suspected that he was up to something. He wasn't. At least, not yet. But soon he would be and he didn't want Carmen to ruin his plans to be with Winnie. It had been a momentous decision for Harry, but he'd come to realise that his happiness lay with Winnie. After all, life was short. This war had shown how precarious life could be. And Harry didn't want to spend the rest of his feeling miserable. But even if he were to live out the rest of his days with Winnie, he knew he couldn't give up his *other* ladies. The ones that saw to his needs but cost him a small fortune. And he hoped that Carmen wouldn't shout her mouth off about them. He doubted that she would as he was sure that Carmen wouldn't want Cheryl to know the truth.

In the Halfway House, the landlord informed Harry that Errol had been in looking for him. Harry worried that something was wrong with Cheryl. He couldn't think of any other reason why Errol would be looking for him. He'd promised Carmen that he wouldn't visit the Battersea Tavern but it was the most likely place for Errol to go and look for him. So Harry chose to have his pint in Winnie's pub instead.

As he made his way there, he was eager to see Winnie.

He'd missed her but he wouldn't tell her of his plans yet. That wouldn't be fair to Carmen. Considering Carmen had been his wife for many years, she at least deserved the respect of being the first to know that he was leaving her.

As he turned the corner, he saw Errol coming out of the pub and he called after him.

Errol offered no smile. When Harry greeted him, he could see only an unnerving fury behind Errol's eyes.

'Wotcha, Son. Everything all right? I hear you've been looking for me.'

'I ain't your son.'

Harry chose to ignore Errol's remark and he went on to say, 'Me and your mum have moved into a new house today. I'll scribble down the address for you. Perhaps you could pass it on to Cheryl? I know your mother would love to see you both.'

'I ain't doing your bidding. If you want Cheryl to know where to find you, you can tell her yourself. You know she's living with my gran.'

'Yeah, all right. I was only asking.'

'Well, don't,' Errol spat.

Harry's heart began to race. He didn't like feeling nervous of the man he'd raised as his own son. But Errol's temper could be unpredictable and it was clear that he had a bee in his bonnet about something. 'Why was you looking for me?' he asked, trying to keep his voice steady.

'To warn you to stay off my turf. I'm selling round here now. Your old customers are coming to me for what they want. And your suppliers are selling to me an' all.'

'W-what are you on about?' Harry spluttered.

'You heard. Stay away!' Errol hissed in his face.

'You can't take over my patch,' Harry protested, panic rising.

'I can and I have. It's only because you're Cheryl's dad that I ain't giving you a good pasting.'

'Please, Errol, don't be like that. I've always done me best for you.'

'It ain't about me. What you and my mother did to Gran is the lowest of the low. You had no scruples. You've taught me well. So well, in fact, that I ain't got any bad feelings about taking over *your* business.'

'But, Errol, you—'

'Piss off, *Dad*,' Errol growled.

Harry found himself shaking, partly in fear of Errol and partly in anger and frustration. He dared not defy Errol and knew that he couldn't fight him. But the business was Harry's livelihood. He needed the income to pay for Carmen's flashy new house. And he couldn't move into Winnie's without any coins jingling in his pockets. 'Your mother will be disappointed in you,' Harry said sadly.

'Yeah. Go tell someone who cares.'

Harry, feeling defeated, looked pleadingly at the man he'd always thought of as his son. But Errol glared back coldly.

With nothing more to say, Harry reluctantly sloped off back home. His mind turned. Where would he earn his money now? Could he buy and sell outside of Battersea? How would Carmen react? Harry decided that until he had worked it all out, it was probably best to keep his wife in the dark for now. After all, he could do without her nagging at him as well.

23

On Sunday afternoon, Cheryl had spent a while helping Yvonne to get ready and had taken even longer over her own appearance. She was more nervous about her date with Bobby than she was letting on. And now Yvonne seemed equally as anxious about meeting Bobby's friend. But, as usual, Yvonne managed to bring the conversation round to Errol.

'What's your dad going to do now that your brother has taken over his business?' Yvonne asked quietly.

'I don't know and I don't care. I'm just glad that Errol didn't kick his head in. I thought he was going to. I've been worried sick about it all week.'

'I wish I had a brother like yours who looked out for me.'

'No you don't, Yvonne. Trust me, he can make things very awkward. I'm not looking forward to Bobby meeting Errol again. It was awful last week, I felt so sorry for Bobby.'

'Errol couldn't have put him off that much, not if he's coming back for more.'

'And with his friend,' Cheryl added, smiling. 'I wonder what he'll be like.'

'Nothing like Errol,' Yvonne mumbled under her breath.

'Anyway, tell me what's been going on in Battersea. Any more gossip about Mrs Berry's son? Have the police found him yet?'

'No, not as far as I know. I still feel terrible. I should have told Mrs Berry about Lucy and David when you asked me too. If I had of done, perhaps the girl would still be alive.'

'It's not your fault, Yvonne. And who's to say that it would have made any difference. Let's face it, I knew about them seeing each other too and I never went out of my way to go to Battersea and tell Mrs Berry. We could all blame ourselves for having some part in Lucy's death but we shouldn't. It wasn't our fault.'

'Yeah, you're right. Poor Mrs Berry has had a rough time lately, what with that and her husband being killed. Though Anne reckons that Mrs Berry doesn't seem too upset about it.'

'I don't blame her. I heard he was a right pig. Right, all done, I'm ready. Come on.'

'You both look smashing,' Edie said when they came downstairs and walked into the front room. Even Errol looked at them approvingly.

'Thanks,' Cheryl said. 'Do you like how I've waved Yvonne's hair?'

'It looks a treat. Bobby and his friend are lucky chaps to have two beauties out with 'em.'

'Thanks, Gran.'

Edie wagged her finger at Errol. 'You remember what I said? Don't go scaring them off. Bobby is a nice lad. Cheryl could do a lot worse.'

Errol smiled warmly at his gran. 'Don't worry. I'll be polite.'

'You'd better be,' Cheryl added. 'I don't want a repeat

of last time. In fact, when they call, I think we should get straight off.'

'Not so fast, young lady. I'd like to meet Bobby's friend too. Whilst Yvonne is here in my house, she's my responsibility.'

'Yvonne isn't living with us, Gran. She only came to stay for the weekend.'

'Makes no odds. I'm sure that Yvonne's mother would be happy to know that I'm vetting the fella.'

Yvonne and Cheryl exchanged a glance and Yvonne said shyly, 'Thanks, Mrs Hampton.'

'They're here!' Cheryl exclaimed. She'd seen two smart-looking blokes walk past the window. And then there was a knock on the door.

'Go and answer it, then,' Edie said, rolling her eyes.

'Come with me, Yvonne.'

'There won't be room in my passageway. Just go and answer the door, stop being so silly. It's only Bobby, not King George.'

Cheryl swallowed hard and then looked excitedly at Yvonne. But Yvonne had her eyes on Errol. She hoped that Bobby's friend would turn Yvonne's head.

At the door, Cheryl showed the young men in and, to her delight, Bobby didn't seem to be in the least bit deterred by Errol's presence.

'Hello, Errol, Yvonne, Mrs Hampton. This is my friend, Ken.'

'It's nice to meet you, Ken. What do you do?' Edie asked.

'I'm a brickie. And the way things are going, if Hitler keeps bombing us, with all the rebuilding that's going to happen, I'll have work coming out of me earholes for life.'

'Well, aren't you the optimist! But it's nice that you can see the good in a bad situation. Where are you taking the ladies?'

Ken shifted from one foot to the other as Bobby answered, 'To Ken's mum's boss's house. Ken's mum is a housekeeper at a big house near the little common. The owners are out of town and have been for months. Ken's mum said we can go round there and use their projector screen. There's nothing open and it's too cold to go for much of a walk. If that's all right with you, Mrs Hampton?'

'There'd better not be any funny business,' Errol barked.

'No, nothing like that. You can come with us, if you like?'

Errol didn't answer but Cheryl saw him wink at their gran.

'It sounds lovely,' Cheryl enthused. 'Shall we get going?'

'Yes. We'll have Cheryl and Yvonne home by seven,' Bobby assured Edie.

'By six,' Errol added and glared threateningly at Bobby.

It took them about twenty minutes to reach the grand house. Cheryl was pleased to see that Yvonne and Ken seemed to be rubbing along together nicely. In fact, Cheryl had never heard Yvonne be so talkative, especially with a fella. 'Are you sure we're allowed in here?' she asked Bobby.

'Yep. As long as we leave the place as we found it.'

Inside, Cheryl and Yvonne gawped at the high ceilings and richly decorated walls. Cheryl felt nervous about knocking over any of the expensive-looking vases. This was just the sort of house her mother would have loved to own. Opulent and extravagant and very ostentatious. She wondered how her mum was. She'd wanted to ask Errol but not in front of her gran. Bringing her mind back to the room, as she gazed at the heavy curtains and lavish paintings, she asked in awe, 'Who owns this place?'

'A barrister and his missus. Ken's mum has been cleaning for 'em for years. But they've gone up to their country home in Scotland and ain't likely to be back until the Germans stop sending bombers over.'

'Is it all right to sit on the sofa?' Yvonne asked.

'Yeah. Make yourself at home,' Ken answered. 'Me and Bobby will get you both drinks. Do you want a sherry?'

'Sherry?' Cheryl blurted. 'Do I look like I'm fifty years old? No, thanks. But we'll have a gin, if there's any?'

Yvonne shot Cheryl a concerned glance.

'There's just about any drink you can think of,' Bobby replied.

While Bobby and Ken went to fetch the drinks, Cheryl wandered over to a piano. 'It's ages since I've had a tinkle,' she said and opened the lid. 'One good thing my mum did for me was to get me piano lessons.' Cheryl sat on the stool and began to play a few notes. The piano sounded perfectly tuned, not that she was an expert.

'You play well,' Bobby said. 'Gin and tonic water,' he added, offering her the glass.

Cheryl sipped the drink and tried not to wrinkle her nose or pull a face at the disgusting flavour. It didn't taste anything like she'd expected but she didn't want to appear unsophisticated in front of Bobby.

Ken had given Yvonne a drink but Cheryl noticed that her friend hadn't drunk hers. Bobby took the glass from Cheryl's hand and placed it on a side table. Then he told her to shimmy over and he sat beside her on the stool. He began tapping on the keys, playing a familiar tune.

'Join in,' he told Cheryl.

She picked up the rhythm and they played in harmony. Yvonne and Ken came to stand beside the piano. Cheryl saw

Ken slip his arm around Yvonne's waist. She thought that they looked good together, like a couple.

'That was fun,' Cheryl said to Bobby after they'd finished playing the music. 'Where did you learn to play the piano?'

'My granddad taught me. We've got a small old piano in the front room but since my granddad passed away, it's mostly used as a sideboard now. My granddad used to tell me about the times that my nan wanted to chop up his piano and use it as firewood when they were too skint to afford coal. It was nice playing with you; it brought back some special memories.'

'That's lovely,' Cheryl said sadly. She didn't have those special memories of her grandparents, thanks to her mum and dad for robbing her of them. Though she was still angry with them, she wanted to see them, especially her dad. She'd always been a daddy's girl and missed being spoiled by him. She walked over to the table and picked up her drink. She managed to get a good few mouthfuls down and found that the taste was becoming more bearable. 'What's this projector thing that you mentioned?' she asked.

'It's in the other room. It's all set up, ready to go.'

'You'd better get me another drink, then,' Cheryl said. She knocked back what was left in her glass and held it aloft to Bobby.

'Hey, slow down. I can't take you back to your gran's drunk.'

'He's right, Cheryl,' Yvonne said. 'Errol will kill him.'

'Spoilsports. Two drinks won't get me drunk.' Though in truth, Cheryl was already feeling a bit giddy.

'All right, I'll get you another but drink it slowly this time,' Bobby said.

In the projector room, Cheryl sat down a seat away from Yvonne, leaving a space for Ken to sit beside her friend. When Bobby joined them and handed her the refilled glass, she purred, 'This is very cosy.'

'Sit tight and I'll get the film rolling.'

Bobby turned out the lights and after a few moments, black-and-white moving images began to flicker on a white screen in front of them.

'It's just like being at the cinema,' Yvonne said, sounding thrilled.

Bobby took hold of Cheryl's hand as they watched an old film of Charlie Chaplin and his funny antics. By the time the short film had finished, so had Cheryl's drink.

'Can we watch another one?' Yvonne asked.

'Sure. Just give me a minute to put another reel on,' Bobby answered.

Cheryl thought that now was a good time to pop to the toilet. But as she started to stand up, she staggered sideways, half falling onto Ken. 'Whoops, sorry,' she said and giggled.

'You're drunk,' Bobby moaned, the disappointment in his voice clear to hear.

'Am I?'

'Yes, you are. No more gin for you or your gran won't let me take you out again.'

Cheryl sidled up to Bobby, placed her arm over his shoulder and leaned into him. 'Would you like to take me out again?' she asked, trying to sound sexy.

'Yeah, I would.' Bobby smiled and gently pushed her away. 'But next time, we'll avoid any booze.'

'I don't feel well,' Cheryl groaned, suddenly feeling the urge to throw up. 'Where's the toilet?' she asked as she ran towards the door. But before anyone could answer, vomit rose in her throat and she leaned forward, chucking up on the floor. 'Oh no, I'm so sorry,' she said sheepishly, cringing inside.

Yvonne rushed to her side. 'Sit down. I'll get you a glass of water.'

'And I'll clean this mess up,' Bobby added.

'No, wait, please, Bobby. I'll clean it,' Cheryl said, her cheeks flaming red.

'No, you just concentrate on feeling better. Leave this to me.'

Yvonne led Cheryl through to the living room and sat beside her on the sofa.

'I'm so embarrassed. I can't believe I did that,' Cheryl whispered.

'Bobby doesn't seem to mind.'

'I bet he does. He'll never want to see me again now!' Cheryl hadn't realised that Bobby had come into the room with a glass of water for her.

'Yes, I will. So whatever silly notion you've got in your head, get it out. I'd love to see you again, Cheryl. Now, drink up.'

Cheryl sipped the water gratefully and immediately began to feel a little better. She'd learned her lesson. There was nothing grown up or sophisticated about swigging gin. And in future, the next time she was out with Bobby, she wouldn't try to show off!

Harry was fast becoming disheartened. So far, four of his suppliers had refused to sell to him or they had offered him ridiculously high prices. Errol had done a good job of stitching him up and now Harry's coffers were almost empty. *The ungrateful swine*, thought Harry, thinking of the money he'd spent on raising Errol. But Harry held more hope of success with Walter. After all, Walter had been his mate since school.

He ambled into Walter's garage, hoping that he'd receive a friendly welcome.

'Wotcha, mate,' Harry said, keeping his voice light.

The instant that Walter lifted his head from under a car bonnet, Harry knew from his friend's expression that Errol had already nobbled him.

'Harry, er, hello. I weren't expecting you.'

'No, I bet you weren't. I suppose you're going to tell me the same as everyone else?'

'What's that, mate?'

'That you ain't got nothing to sell or else you'll offer me over-inflated prices.'

'See, the thing is, mate—'

'Don't bother, Walter. This ain't the first time that you've let me down.'

'I didn't have any choice. You know how *persuasive* your Errol can be.'

'Did he threaten you?' Harry seethed.

'Not directly but we both know how he works. What was I supposed to do, eh? You tell me.'

Harry sighed heavily. 'He's a scheming git. He's done me up like a kipper, Walter.'

'Sorry to hear that, mate. What are you going to do about it?'

'I don't know. But if I don't do something soon, me and the missus will be on the streets.'

Walter went towards a metal cupboard, wiping his hands

on his overalls. He then pulled out a tin and took a couple of pound notes out. ' 'Ere. It ain't much but I hope it helps.'

Harry looked horrified at the offer. 'No, Walter, I don't want your handouts!'

'Just take it, mate.'

Harry couldn't bring himself to answer Walter or to take the money. He turned on his heel and marched out, feeling ashamed that his friend had felt compelled to offer him charity. It had been bad enough that he'd accepted help from Winnie and had stayed in her home but at least he'd been able to more than pay his way. But this! And his feeling of shame was made worse by the knowledge that he was almost destitute.

The streets were quiet, a typical Sunday evening. Harry was on the other side of Battersea and had to face a long and lonely walk home. He didn't rush. There was no joy in thinking of the greeting he'd receive from Carmen. His wife would be waiting with her arm outstretched and her hand open, ready for him to put cash into it. But he had nothing to give her. He'd be left with no option other than to tell her the truth. That wasn't a thought to relish. Carmen was already upset about not seeing Cheryl and Errol. He'd have to explain to her that they were skint because of her precious son and would likely lose the house because Errol had stolen their income. She wouldn't take the news well and he'd be left to put up with her mood. The thought left him wanting to run into Winnie's arms. But he couldn't. Not yet. Not until he could provide Carmen with a home and offer Winnie at least his keep. Gawd, it was grim.

Harry dragged his feet and was deep in thought. He really didn't want to go home. He was wallowing in self-pity but he found the peace on the empty streets somewhat comforting. It was better than having Carmen mithering in his ear. The stillness and quietness of the evening was suddenly disturbed by the sound of Moaning Minnie wailing into life. Christ, the racket was as bad as Carmen's whining! All at once, the sky was illuminated with searchlights and the incoming hum of enemy aircraft could clearly be heard.

Harry looked skyward. He couldn't see the planes yet but he could hear that there were many of them. His heart raced. This was going to be a heavy and gruesome attack. *Where are the RAF?* he thought, scanning the sky. He caught sight of the first of the German fighter planes leading the way for dozens of bombers. The formation stretched across the sky for as far as he could see. Stunned by the sight, Harry stood rooted to the spot, gazing despairingly upwards, barely able to comprehend the enormity of what he could see.

An explosion pricked his ears. It was several streets away but too close for comfort. Another one, closer this time. Fires crackled into life as incendiaries began to land. Harry knew that he wasn't safe where he stood. But what could he do? He looked along the street. Rows and rows of terraced houses in both directions with a large bakery in the middle.

BOOM! Harry ran. He couldn't see where the bomb had landed but a cloud of smoke rose upwards from the end of the street. The noise was deafening and Harry found he was struggling to breathe, his lungs thick with brick dust. BOOM! Another explosion. It lifted Harry off his feet. He felt himself flying through the air and he screamed in agony as an incredible heat engulfed his body and seared his skin. He landed somewhere with a terrific thump, singed and blackened, hardly feeling the twisted piece of metal that pierced his chest.

Harry coughed and spluttered, gasping desperately for air. He lay on his back, spreadeagled and impaled on the ground by the shard of metal and a heavy lump of concrete. He could feel his skin blistering and he cried in pain. 'Help … me …' His plea was just a soft croak, lost in the sound of the snapping fires and thunderous explosions. He thought of Cheryl and feared he'd never see her again. Winnie would never know that he loved her.

The light from a torch shone in his eyes, momentarily blinding him.

'Is he alive?' a voice asked.

'It's not looking good. He's burned to a crisp. I don't think he's going to make it,' another said grimly.

Harry felt the crippling pain leave his charred and broken body. A feeling of overwhelming tranquillity washed over him. The world fell silent and the light from the torch seemed to get brighter and brighter, engulfing every part of him and filling him with love. He found himself feeling as though he was floating upwards. Floating in the light. Harry had found his peace. Forever.

24

London had been battered night after night by the Luftwaffe but Sunday night's attack had been the worst so far. On Monday morning, Winnie stood behind the bar and wanted to cover her ears so that she wouldn't have to listen to any more heart-wrenching stories from her customers. But at least St Paul's Cathedral had been saved. An army of firemen and volunteers had bravely guarded the place all night and had extinguished the incendiaries and infernos that threatened the iconic landmark. The papers and the wireless were full of it. St Paul's dome had been saved! *But what about all the rest of the poor bleeders who'd lost their homes and loved ones*, Winnie thought sadly as she tried to put a brave face on her woes.

She looked up from the newspaper on the bar and saw Carmen storm in and stamp across the pub, her eyes blaring with anger.

'Where is he?' Carmen screeched.

'Who?' Winnie asked though she could guess that Carmen was referring to Harry.

'You know full well who! Where is my husband?'

Before Winnie could claim that she had no idea where

Harry was, Bernie rushed in. He was normally rosy-cheeked, as he was always darting around, but, this morning, he looked as white as the sheet that was still wrapped around his injured head. Winnie could see that the man was shaken. Ignoring Carmen, she asked Bernie urgently, 'What's wrong?'

'It's the bakery, Win. It's been blown up!'

'Oh, blimey! Thank Gawd Terry's away at basic training and weren't in there!'

'Yeah, good job he signed up, but you'll never guess who was nearby? Have-it Harry. He was caught up in the explosion. He's dead, Win.'

Winnie stared at Bernie but no words would form on her lips.

'What did you just say?' Carmen asked slowly.

Bernie looked over to see Carmen.

'God, I'm sorry, Mrs Hampton, I didn't see you there.'

'Did you say that Harry is dead? My husband Harry?'

After a painful pause, Bernie answered. 'Yes. I'm so sorry.'

Winnie hadn't realised, but tears were falling freely down her cheeks.

'What are you crying for? He was *my* husband!' Carmen screamed.

Rachel spoke up for Winnie. 'She's probably been reminded that her husband was killed just recently too.'

'Huh, her tears ain't for her husband! She's crying for *mine*. Go on, admit it, Winnie. You're upset because the man, who you openly had an affair with right under my nose, is dead. Well, cry your bleedin' heart out cos now you'll never have him. Never!'

It was true, well, most of it. Winnie's tears were for Harry. She couldn't deny it. But she wouldn't stand there and allow

Carmen to sully Harry's memory. 'I'm sorry for your loss but I've told you before that there was nothing going on with me and Harry. You're not welcome in my pub, so sling your spiteful arse out. NOW!'

'You're disgusting,' Carmen said. She spat on the floor before marching out.

'I need a minute,' Winnie whispered to Rachel.

Upstairs, Winnie threw herself onto her bed and sobbed into her pillow. She knew she had no right to mourn Harry, he wasn't her husband. But, rightly or wrongly, she'd loved the man. And now he was gone along with all her dreams.

Cheryl came out from the stockroom and was stunned to find Errol in the shop. 'What are you doing here?' she asked.

'I've come to take you to Gran's for lunch. When is your break?'

'In ten minutes. Why are you taking me to Gran's?'

'I'll tell you when we get there. I'll wait outside.'

Errol ambled off leaving Cheryl wondering what he was up to. It seemed very odd for him to have come over to Balham just to take her home for lunch. He was obviously hiding something from her. Cheryl's stomach knotted at the thought of bad news.

Another shop assistant walked over to Cheryl. 'Was that your fella?' Maureen asked.

'No, my brother.'

'He's a bit of all right. Has he got a girlfriend?'

'Er, yeah,' Cheryl answered. Her eyes narrowed as she looked through the window at Errol outside smoking a cigarette. What was he up to?

Ten minutes later, Errol walked Cheryl to his mate's car.

'I've bought this from Tommo,' he said, pointing at the vehicle.

'You must be doing well with Dad's business.'

'Can't complain. Get in,' he said.

'What's going on, Errol? Why have you driven over?'

'I've told you, wait till we're at Gran's.'

Cheryl huffed. She didn't like surprises and she hated being kept in the dark.

'It's only us,' she called as she opened her gran's front door. 'Errol is with me.'

In the front room, Edie beamed at Errol. 'Hello, dear, what a lovely surprise. What brings you here today? I wasn't expecting you until the weekend.'

'I've come for a cuppa, Gran. I'm gasping,' Errol answered.

'You've come a long way from Battersea just for a cuppa,' Edie chuckled. 'It's a good job that I've got some of your favourite biscuits left from yesterday. Hang on, I'll get them for you.'

'No, it's all right, Gran, stay there.'

'I'll fetch them and I'll make the tea,' Cheryl offered.

When she came back into the front room carrying a tray, Errol jumped up from the sofa to take it from her. Something wasn't right, Cheryl could sense it. Errol seemed out of sorts and she had the feeling that there was something he wanted to say. 'Why are you really here?' she asked.

Errol looked into his teacup and then his eyes met hers. 'There's no easy way of saying this, so I'll come straight out with it. I've come to tell you that during the bombing last night, your dad was killed.'

Cheryl gasped and her gran cried out, 'No … no! That can't be right. Harry can't be dead. He can't be! Are you sure?'

'Yes, Gran, I'm sorry but I'm sure.'

Cheryl had a thousand thoughts spinning around in her mind but she couldn't speak.

Edie wept and shook her head. 'It ain't right. It ain't right. That's both my boys killed in wars. A mother shouldn't have to outlive her sons. It ain't right.'

'No, it's not. I feel for you, Gran, I really do,' Errol said. He looked at Cheryl and asked, 'Are you all right, Sis?'

Cheryl, her lips pursed, nodded.

'You're not, are you?' he pushed.

This time, Cheryl shook her head.

Errol moved along the sofa and put his arm across her. 'Don't worry, I'll always look after you.'

Cheryl, feeling numb, looked over to her gran who was blowing her nose into a handkerchief. She wanted to comfort the old lady but she didn't know what to say. No words could take away her pain. How can comfort be offered to a woman who has lost both her children?

Edie sniffed and between crying breaths, she said, 'I suppose Carmen will be arranging his funeral but I'd like Harry buried with his father, my Wilf.'

Cheryl hadn't considered her mother and asked Errol, 'How is Mum?'

'I don't know. I haven't seen her yet.'

'We should go to her.'

'Yeah, we should. Do you want to go now? I can take you.'

'I'm not sure that we should leave Gran,' she whispered.

'I might be old but I ain't deaf. I heard you. Don't be daft, I'll be fine. I've spent years alone; I know how to care for myself. I'm not bothered about your mother but you two should be with her at a time like this. Leave me be.'

'Are you sure, Gran?' Errol asked. 'We won't leave you if you're too upset.'

'I'd rather be alone for a while. Just me and my memories. Go on, get off and see your mother. I've lost a husband, so I understand the pain she must be feeling.'

Cheryl climbed into Errol's car and looked back at her gran's neat little house. The poor old woman was inside breaking her heart. She hated to leave her gran to grieve alone. But her mother was alone too.

Errol turned the engine and they set off to Battersea. Cheryl dreaded to think what state they'd find their mother in. She took a deep breath but didn't have to stop herself from crying. It didn't feel real. Maybe it would when she got back to Battersea. 'I haven't told Mr Mapleford that I'm not coming back after lunch.'

'Don't worry, your manager will understand.'

'What's Mum's new house like?' Cheryl asked.

'Dunno. I ain't been there.'

Cheryl soon saw for herself. The house looked bigger than their family home had been and was in a nicer part of Battersea. 'Dad did well,' Cheryl said, and then the agonising sadness hit her. Her throat felt tight, as did her chest. She knew it was because she was holding in her sorrow.

They stood side by side on the doorstep and Errol knocked on the door. There was no answer, so he knocked again, heavier, louder. When there was still no reply, Cheryl called through the letterbox. 'Mum ... Mum ... It's us, me and Errol.'

She saw a shadowy figure come into the passageway and then her mother opened the door. Cheryl could see that her mum's black eye make-up was intact and there was no visible puffiness around her eyes. It didn't look like the woman had shed a single tear.

'You've heard about your father, then?'

'Yes, Mum.'

'It's decent of you to show your faces. You'd better come in.'

Cheryl and Errol followed their mother through to the kitchen where Carmen lit the gas under the kettle. 'I've no sugar and the tea will be weak. I've only used leaves left. And I can't make you a sandwich or anything.'

Cheryl went to the larder and opened the door. She was shocked to find her mother's cupboards bare. 'Why haven't you got any food in?'

'I'm skint. Your father hadn't given me a bean before he died and he's left me with nothing.'

'Oh, Mum, you can't live like this. You've got to eat,' Cheryl said. She rummaged in her handbag for her purse but Errol put his hand on her arm.

'I'll see to Mum,' he said quietly. He pulled a wad of notes from his pocket and then peeled off several which he placed on the kitchen table. 'That should see you through for a while.'

Their mother looked scathingly at them. 'I'm so ashamed. Never in my life have I had to accept handouts. And from me own kids an' all. This is your father's fault!'

Cheryl glared at Errol. It wasn't her father's fault that their mother had no money. It was Errol's fault. He'd taken her dad's business and left her parents with nothing.

'I won't see you starve, Mum,' Errol assured.

'What about the rent on this place? Are you going to pay that too?'

'I can help with that, Mum, but you don't need a big house like this. We'll find you a nice little flat, somewhere closer to mine, eh?'

'A flat! I'm not living in a flat! I feel like I'm going backwards in life, thanks to your useless father!'

'Please don't talk about my dad like that,' Cheryl requested sadly. 'He made a lot of mistakes in his life but he's dead. Show him some respect.'

'Don't come into my home and tell me what I can and cannot say about your father. I'll speak as I find and as I like. Your father was useless, that's a fact! He was a womaniser an' all. If you don't believe me, go and ask Winnie Berry.'

'What's Winnie Berry got to do with anything?' Cheryl asked.

'Her and your father were at it, that's what! He was probably throwing his money at her too, showing off like he did, and that's why I ain't seen a penny.'

Errol roared with laughter.

'What's so funny?' Carmen asked.

'Harry and Mrs Berry? I think you're way off the mark there, Mum. But you're right; he was useless and had no spine. He earned enough money over the years to buy you this house and more besides. But he squandered it on flash clothes and playing at being the big man. And you're as bad, having to have the best of everything. Neither of you bothered to put any money by and now look at the mess you're in.'

'Who do you think you are, Errol Hampton? You know nothing of my business. For your information, I had plenty put by, thank you very much. Why do you think our curtains were so heavy? It's because I'd sown me savings into them but they went up in smoke when the house was bombed.

So don't you dare put me in the same category as your good-for-nothing father!'

'He wasn't my father, though, was he, Mum? I was just a dirty secret that you were both ashamed of. But I'm glad he weren't my dad and I'm sorry that you're my mother.'

'Stop it!' Cheryl shouted. 'Please, stop it! My dad is dead. You both might have hated him but I loved him.' The tears that Cheryl had held back began to fall in a rushing cascade. Her thick sobs wracked her body.

'Sit down,' Errol said softly.

He pulled out a seat at the kitchen table but Cheryl had no desire to stay in the house with her hateful mother. She wanted her dad to comfort her. But he couldn't and he never would again. 'I want to go home,' she cried.

'Yeah, that's right. You bugger off back to your gran. She hasn't seen your father in years but I bet her crocodile tears are falling while she's demanding sympathy for her dead son.'

Errol shot his mother an angry look. 'Come on, Sis. Let's leave her to wallow in her own nastiness.' He gently urged Cheryl towards the door and then turned back to his mum. 'I'll find you somewhere to live and I'll make sure you've got money. But I'm only doing it because it's the right thing to do. To be honest, Mum, you don't deserve it.'

In the car, Cheryl's shoulders shook as she cried. 'I hate her, Errol,' she said through juddering breaths. 'She's so horrid about everyone.'

'She's grieving and she's worried about money. You know what she's like; Mum shows her upset through anger. I reckon she's only got two emotions, anger and bitterness.'

'She's not grieving! The only thing Mum cares about is money. I don't think she even cares about us.'

'She does, Sis, especially you. She thinks the world of you but she's just got a funny way of showing it.'

Cheryl didn't agree with her brother and thought that Errol was being too charitable about their mother. She felt terrible for thinking it but Cheryl wished it was her mum who had been killed instead of her dad. Her dear dad. She'd been so annoyed with him. If only she'd made amends with him sooner. Now it was too late and Cheryl knew that she'd spend the rest of her life regretting it.

25

'I think we should have a get-together here in memory of Harry. I can put on a bit of a spread and we can all raise a glass to him.'

'That's a lovely idea, Win,' Rachel agreed.

'Carmen hasn't organised anything for him and Harry was ever such a popular bloke, I think folk need to do something to mark his passing.'

'I can make some posters, if you like, to get word out?'

'No, thanks, Rachel, I don't think that's the done thing. We can tell our customers. Word will spread. We'll hold it on Saturday morning.'

'That's only two days away. Is that enough time to organise everything?'

'Yes, I think so,' Winnie answered. 'But I'll check with Errol before we invite anyone.'

'Talk of the devil,' Rachel said as Errol walked in.

'Hello, ladies. My usual, please. I must say, Mrs Berry, you're looking very well today.'

'Thanks, love. I wish I felt it. But I'm as worn out as the rest of us,' Winnie answered. Since Errol had been conducting his business in her pub, she'd been pleased that he'd stuck to his word and hadn't stepped out of line. He didn't even leer at Rachel anymore. 'How are you?' she asked.

'As fresh as a daisy. I sleep right through the air raids. The way I see it, when your time's up, your time's up.'

'You're braver than me. I try and get my head down but I can't say that my sleep is restful.'

Rachel placed his drink on the bar but before Errol walked over to his table, Winnie asked, 'Can I have a word?'

'Always, Mrs Berry. You can have as many words as you like.'

'I was thinking that it might be nice to hold a bit of a do in here on Saturday morning in memory of your dad. What do you think?'

Errol scowled. 'Do what you want. But I don't want any part of it.'

'Oh, I'm sorry, love. I won't if you'd rather I didn't?'

'Like I said, do what you want. I don't suppose my mother will arrange much of a send-off for him.'

'How is she?'

'Same as always.'

'She's probably told you that I've thrown her out of here but she's welcome to come on Saturday. Will you let her know?'

'Yeah, but don't hold your breath.'

'Thanks, love. I've made some pork pies with that meat you gave me yesterday. Would you like one with a nice bit of pickle?'

The smile returned to Errol's face as he answered, 'I wouldn't say no, Mrs Berry.'

'Go and sit yourself down, I'll bring it over.'

Winnie went through to the back kitchen thinking about the conversation she'd had with Errol. She couldn't understand why he was so cold towards Harry. It must have been an awful argument that they'd had. She thought it was sad that father and son hadn't sorted their differences before Harry had died. Winnie swallowed hard as she fought to stop herself from blubbering again. She'd cried herself to sleep for the past three nights. Harry had no idea of the pain he'd left behind.

As Winnie spooned pickle onto a plate, she heard raised voices coming from the bar. She left the plate on the side and rushed out to see what all the commotion was about.

When she walked in, Winnie saw Errol roughly handling three soldiers. He was throwing them out of the pub. One was holding a bloodied nose and the other two were helping to hold him up.

'I've only been gone two minutes. What the hell happened?' Winnie asked. She looked from Rachel to Errol for an answer.

It was Rachel who explained. 'Those three came in being right lairy and the one who's now got a broken nose said something very unsavoury that I won't repeat! So Errol jumped in, lumped him one and threw them out. Good job that Errol did or I would have given that cheeky swine a right mouthful!'

'Who'd have thought it, eh? Errol Hampton being the hero in my pub. Thanks, love, you can have a drink on me for that.'

'No need, Mrs Berry. I couldn't sit by and watch them insult Rachel.'

'Good for you. I'll go and get that pork pie.'

Winnie went back into the kitchen feeling somewhat stunned at Errol's valiant conduct. It was one thing for him to behave himself in her pub, but now he was proving himself quite an asset to have around. She just wished that she wasn't reminded of Harry every time she looked at him.

Bobby had one hand on a piece of pork and a cleaver in the other. He was busy cutting the joint into smaller pieces but kept glancing up to look out of the butcher's shop window, hoping to catch a glance of Cheryl passing.

'Watch what you're doing, Bobby, you'll have your fingers off,' the master butcher said.

'Yeah, thanks, Mr Beckett, you're right. I'll be more careful,' Bobby answered. But his mind wasn't on his job. He hadn't seen Cheryl at work for a few days and he was worried that something bad had happened to her.

'I'm guessing it's that pretty little dark-haired lady who has got your attention?'

'Yes, Cheryl. She works over at Barratt's shoe shop, but I've not seen her for a few days. I hope she's all right.'

Mr Beckett, a rotund man with a large red nose, wandered to the shop window and looked up and down the street. 'Do you know where Cheryl lives?'

'Yes, just around the corner from me.'

'Then put us both out of our misery and go and check on her. It's quiet today and I don't suppose it's going to get any busier. I can't have you doing yourself a mischief because you're not concentrating.'

Bobby whipped off his blue-and-white striped apron and removed his straw boater hat before dashing through to the back off the shop. He returned, pulling his coat on as he walked. 'Thanks, Mr Beckett. I'll just check on her and then come straight back to clean up.'

'No, don't worry, lad. I'll see you tomorrow.'

As Bobby hurried out of the door, he heard Mr Beckett call, 'I hope your young lady is all right.'

A short while later, Bobby knocked on Edie's door. He felt uncomfortable calling without an invite and hoped he wasn't imposing. But he was pleased to see Cheryl when she opened the door.

'Bobby! Oh, hello,' she said.

'I hope you don't mind me popping round?'

'No, of course not. But shouldn't you be at work?'

'Yes, but Mr Beckett has given me the rest of the day off. I was worried; I haven't seen you at work for few days.'

Cheryl pulled the door open wider. 'Come in,' she said, looking sad.

'Are you sure?'

'Yes. Something terrible has happened and, to be honest, I could do with a distraction and so could my gran.'

Bobby followed Cheryl into the front room, wondering what was wrong but he didn't like to ask.

'Hello, dear,' Edie greeted but she barely raised a smile.

'I hope I'm not intruding?'

'You're always welcome here. Has she told you?'

'No,' Bobby answered and he looked at Cheryl.

'My dad's dead. He was killed by a bomb.'

'I'm sorry to hear that. You must both be devastated.' Bobby quickly removed his flat cap and fingered it awkwardly. He wished he could find something comforting to say or that he had the nerve to reach out and pull Cheryl into his arms.

'Sit down. Cheryl will get you a cuppa.'

Bobby sat on the edge of the sofa and searched for something to say.

Edie pulled out a faded photograph from her cardigan pocket and held it out to him. 'This was my Harry when he was a few years younger than you. He was a good-looking fella and could charm the flies off a turd.'

Bobby took the photo and studied the image. It wasn't very clear but he could see the family resemblance to Cheryl.

'I hadn't seen Harry in years and years but a mother's love never fades.'

Still unsure of what to say, Bobby was grateful when Cheryl came in with a cup of tea for him.

'I see my gran is being maudlin,' Cheryl said.

'You look like your dad,' Bobby said. He smiled and handed the photograph back to Edie.

'Yes, she does. But she looks more like her mother.'

Cheryl sat beside him but rose to her feet again when there was a knock on the front door.

'Blimey, it's like Clapham Junction station here today,' Edie said and she rolled her eyes.

Cheryl peeked through the net curtains. 'It's Errol,' she said.

Bobby's pulse quickened. Though he tried to brush off Errol's abruptness, he found the man to be intimidating and he wouldn't like to get on the wrong side of him. Bobby would have found an excuse to make a hasty exit but he hadn't yet drunk his tea.

'Hello, Gran – Bobby,' Errol greeted them.

'Hello, Son,' Edie said. She pushed herself out of her chair. 'Cheryl will fetch you a cuppa. I've got some of my special biscuits made for you. Sit down, I'll get them.'

Errol sat on the cane chair and glared at Bobby.

'I'm sorry to hear about your dad. I hadn't seen Cheryl at work so I called in to see if she was all right.'

'He wasn't my dad,' Errol answered solemnly. But then his voice lifted when he added, 'It was good of you to check on my sister.'

'Is there anything I can do?' Bobby offered.

'Yeah, there is. There's a memorial thing for Harry on Saturday morning at a pub in Battersea. You can take Cheryl. Keep an eye on her.'

Bobby nodded. He'd have to ask Mr Beckett for the day off work and Saturdays were their busiest time. But given the circumstances, he was sure that his kind and reasonable boss wouldn't mind too much.

'I can pick you up and bring you back but I won't be staying at the pub,' Errol said.

'Thanks.'

'Pick him up for what?' Cheryl asked. She handed Errol a cup of tea and then Edie came back into the room carrying a plate of biscuits.

'Mrs Berry is putting on a do at the pub on Saturday for your dad. Bobby said he'll go with you. I'll drive you both.'

'And me,' Edie said. 'I'd like to go too. It would be nice to meet the people who thought well of my son.'

'Sure, Gran, you can go too. Harry's friends would love to meet you too,' Errol said warmly.

Bobby was pleasantly surprised to see this softer side of Errol. He'd thought the bloke was nothing more than a thug and a bully but now he could see that there was more to him.

'You don't have to come if you don't want to,' Cheryl said to Bobby. 'I'd understand.'

'I'll be with you. I'd like to be.'

Errol took a biscuit from the plate and Bobby noticed that

his knuckles were cut and swollen. Edie must have spotted it too.

'Who have you been punching?' she asked.

Errol glanced at the back of his hand. 'Some Yank in the pub who was rude to the barmaid. It's nothing, Gran.'

'You're just like your granddad. He was chivalrous like that. He punched a chap's lights out once because he'd patted my backside. Mind you, in them days, I was quite a picture. Not a sagging old girl who's getting as blind as a bat.'

'You're still beautiful, Gran,' Errol said, grinning.

'You've got his gift of the gab an' all.'

'I should get going,' Bobby said. 'But I'll be here on Saturday morning.'

'I thought you had the day off?' Edie quizzed.

'I do. But this is family time.'

'Is Cheryl your girl?' Edie asked.

'I'd like to think so, if she'll have me,' Bobby answered uneasily.

'Then you're family. There's no need to feel awkward or to stand on ceremony around us. Yes, we've had a tragedy in the family, just like hundreds of other families in London at the moment. Stay; Cheryl would like you to.'

'Thank you. I'm honoured.'

'I wouldn't be,' Edie chuckled. 'We're a family with dark secrets.'

'Don't scare him off, Gran,' Errol said. 'There's no one else banging down the door for Cheryl.'

Edie and Errol laughed and Cheryl threw a cushion at her brother.

'It don't feel right to laugh,' Edie sniffed suddenly, her eyes filling with tears. 'My Harry is gone. But life goes on and we have to get on with it, I suppose. I've been sitting in this chair for days doing nothing other than crying me eyes out and feeling sorry for myself. Cheryl's been putting on a brave face but the walls in this house are thin and I've heard her crying herself to sleep. No amount of tears will bring him back.'

'Harry wouldn't have wanted you both to be sad,' Errol said softly. 'He'd want you to laugh, Gran. He enjoyed a good laugh himself.'

'Yeah, you're right, he did,' Cheryl agreed. 'Do you remember some of the jokes he used to play on us when we were kids?'

'Yeah, like when he hid that manikin's head in the larder and sent you to get him a piece of cheese. You screamed the house down,' Errol recalled with a chortle.

Cheryl was laughing now too. 'And when he pretended that you was invisible. He kept it going for days. He made me and Mum pretend that we couldn't see you either. Cor, you was doing your nut, shouting, "I'm here, you must be able to see me." I don't know how we kept a straight face for all that time.'

'Mum didn't always appreciate his humour. Remember when he hid all the cutlery and replaced it with knives, forks and spoons that he'd carved from carrots and parsnips?'

'Oh yes, I remember that. Mum made a stew from the veg and then we had no spoons to eat it with,' Cheryl said, tears of laughter streaming down her face.

Bobby listened intently and was pleased to see them laughing and enjoying their memories. He'd have liked to have met Harry. He sounded like a right character.

'This is how we should think of Harry – with laughter. It's what he would have wanted,' Edie said fondly.

Errol stood up. 'I'll get going now and I'll be back on Saturday to pick you up.' Then he turned to Bobby and offered him his hand.

Bobby, though taken by surprise, jumped to his feet and shook Errol's hand.

'Look after my girls for me,' Errol said.

'I will,' Bobby answered. He felt relieved that Errol had dropped his hard-man act but he would always be cautious of the man.

Cheryl saw Errol out. Alone with Bobby, Edie whispered, 'Cheryl was very close to her father. She's going to need you to help her get through this time.'

'I'll be here for her,' Bobby assured her. He'd only met Cheryl a few times but he was already smitten. He thought about her all the time, usually with a ridiculous smile on his face. It was too soon to say that he wanted to spend the rest of his life with her, but the way Bobby was feeling about his girl, he hoped that one day she would become his wife.

26

Winnie sat on the edge of her bed and looked at herself in the mirror. Today was going to be a tough day to get through without shedding more tears for Harry but she was determined to stay strong. *You can do this*, she told her reflection, *and you'll wear a smile on your face all day.*

She turned her head sideways and looked at the repair to the wardrobe door, where Brian had once put his fist through it. That had been the morning when she'd told him about the daughter she'd given up at birth before they'd been married. Brian had been furious. He'd called her awful names. But at the time, Winnie had found a strength within herself that she hadn't known she had. After years of enduring Brian's brutality, that strength had given her the courage to finally stand up to him. She called on that strength now.

Winnie breathed in deeply before standing up and smoothing down her dress. She pushed her shoulders back and opened her bedroom door with gusto. It wasn't the wake of Harry's funeral but she was going to make sure that he had a send-off to be proud of.

'Rachel, are you ready?' she called.

Rachel emerged from her bedroom dressed in a sombre black dress.

'You can get back in there and change out of that,' Winnie ordered, pointing at Rachel's outfit. 'Today is about celebrating Harry's life.'

'Sorry, Win,' Rachel muttered.

'Hurry up. I'll see you downstairs.'

Winnie walked into the bar, satisfied with how it looked. Food was laid out on the table and she'd dragged out the red, white and blue bunting and hung it over the bar. She thought Harry would have liked it. It was cheerful, just like he had been.

She unlocked the door and returned to stand behind the bar with *that* smile fixed on her face. Hilda was the first to arrive, always early, ready to lend a hand.

'Morning, Winnie. Anything I can do?'

'No, thanks, love, not at the moment. But I suspect it's going to be very busy today, so I'm going to need Rachel behind the bar.'

'Great, that means I get to have my granddaughter all to myself.' Hilda smiled. 'How are you bearing up?'

'So so. I don't know why I'm so upset.'

'Because the man you loved, he died, Win. Love is such a strong emotion and so is grief. Don't be too hard on yourself. You're allowed to be upset.'

'I'm not, though, am I? I'm not allowed to be upset. Harry wasn't mine to love.'

'You and Harry got on like a house on fire. Everyone could see that. He wasn't your husband but he was your friend and you're allowed to love your friends. I love you, there's nothing wrong with that.'

'That's a good way of putting it. Thanks, love. Go upstairs and hurry Rachel along. She's getting dressed but I suspect Martha is holding her up.'

'Will do. I'll stay upstairs but give me a shout if you need me.'

Winnie was proud of how far Hilda had come. She'd once been a foul-mouthed drunk but she'd kept her word to Rachel and hadn't touched a drop of booze for a while now. Sober Hilda had a heart of gold and was a dear friend but Winnie hoped they'd never see drunken Hilda again.

'Morning,' Len said as he arrived. 'The place is looking fine,' he added.

'Thanks, Len. I'm determined we'll keep today a happy one.'

'It's what Harry would have wanted.'

More people flocked in, which kept Winnie and Rachel busy. Winnie caught snippets of conservations about Harry. Everyone spoke fondly of him and the atmosphere was jolly though tinged with sadness. She hadn't noticed Cheryl come in until the girl was at the bar with a chap beside her and an old woman next to him.

'Thanks for doing this for my dad, Mrs Berry. It's smashing to see so many people here.'

'Your father was a popular man, love. Who's this?'

'This is my gran, Edie Hampton, and Bobby, my boyfriend. Bobby, Gran, this is Mrs Berry, the landlady. Me and my friends from the factory used to come in here after work. Mrs Berry always looked after us.'

'Nice to meet you both. What can I get you to drink?'

'No gin for me today,' Cheryl whispered to Bobby. 'Just a lemonade.'

'A lemonade for Cheryl, a sherry for Edie and a half for me, thank you,' he said, pointing to one of the pumps.

Winnie got their drinks but wouldn't accept payment. 'I insist,' she told Bobby.

Piano Pete arrived. 'Do you want me to play a few tunes?' he asked.

'Not yet, love. Maybe later. I think we should have a toast to Harry first and someone should say a few words. Do you want to say something, Cheryl?'

'No, I don't think I can. But you should. You and my dad were good friends. And you've done this for him.'

'I don't think it's my place to say something,' Winnie protested. She scanned the bar, searching for someone in the crowd who'd be better placed to talk about Harry.

'Please, Mrs Berry. It would mean a lot to me if you said something.'

'And to me,' Edie added.

Winnie felt awkward but reluctantly agreed. 'All right, I'll say a few words but I'll keep it brief.' She hadn't planned on giving a speech and hoped she wouldn't crack and show her emotions.

She rang the bell to get everyone's attention. Her mouth suddenly felt very dry and her heart raced. Once the pub had fallen silent, and when all eyes were on her, Winnie took a deep breath and then said loudly, 'Thank you for coming today. We're here to remember Harry Hampton, or *Have-it* Harry, as most of us knew him by. Cheryl, his daughter, and his mother, Edie, have asked me to say a few words about him. But let's be honest, Harry could never be summed up in just a few words. He was a larger-than-life character who touched many lives, who brought fun and laughter wherever he went. His smile and banter—'

Winnie was interrupted by the sound of someone slowly clapping. Heads turned to look at where it was coming from. And then the small crowd parted as Carmen walked towards the bar.

Winnie had invited the woman out of politeness but she hadn't expected Carmen to show up. Especially as it was known that she hadn't bothered to organise any kind of gathering or reception after Harry's funeral.

'Very nice speech about *my* husband,' Carmen said sarcastically. 'Sorry, I didn't mean to interrupt. Do carry on.'

Winnie glared at Carmen and she could feel her cheeks reddening. She hoped that the woman wouldn't shout out her accusations about the supposed affair. And now Winnie didn't feel at all comfortable about continuing her words for Harry. 'Maybe you'd like to say something?' she asked Carmen.

'Yes, I would.' Carmen turned to face Winnie's customers.

Winnie dreaded to think what Carmen was about to say and she wanted to run and hide. But she couldn't, so, instead, she braced herself.

'You can forget about attending Harry's funeral because I've already had him buried. Don't look so shocked. Don't pretend that you care. Not one of you has called round to see how I am. Half of you today have only turned up for the free grub. None of you really knew Harry. You might think that you did but you don't have a clue about him. Good old Have-it Harry Hampton, always up for a laugh. Well, it ain't so funny to be left a penniless widow. That's right, penniless because—'

'*Shut your poisonous mouth!*' Edie shouted.

Winnie was astonished that such a loud noise could come out of a frail-looking old woman. But she was pleased that Edie had spoken up.

Edie pushed past Cheryl and walked up to Carmen and stared at her as though she had a bad smell under her nose. Everyone seemed to be holding their breath and waiting for what Edie was going to say next. But instead of giving Carmen a mouthful, a gasp went around the pub when Edie slapped Carmen across the cheek.

'You took my son from me. I won't allow you to take his dignity. Get out, you hateful woman.'

Carmen held her hand to her cheek and looked as though she was going to say something to Edie. But she didn't and Winnie was pleased to see Carmen march off.

The customers began mumbling between themselves, clearly shocked at what they'd witnessed. Winnie rang the bell again and the pub fell quiet. She held a glass of sherry aloft. 'To Harry,' she said. 'He brightened our lives but now may he rest in peace.'

'To Harry,' people parroted.

Winnie looked over at Cheryl; she was crying but she was being comforted by Bobby. The poor girl. What an awful way to find out that her father had already been buried. And now his farewell do had been ruined by Carmen and Harry's name had been soiled. Carmen had said she'd been left penniless, which Winnie found difficult to believe. The woman couldn't be *that* skint, living in such a big house.

'Thank you for what you were saying about my son,' Edie said. 'It's a shame that his widow came in and spoiled it.'

Winnie was just grateful that her name hadn't been brought into Carmen's speech. She hoped she'd seen the back of that vile woman forever.

'I can't believe that my mum had my dad's funeral without me,' Cheryl sobbed once they'd returned home to Edie's house. 'How could she do something like that?'

'She's wicked. She deprived me of my son for all those years and now she's deprived me of saying a proper goodbye to him,' Edie said.

'Losing my dad got me thinking and I realised that I should have it made up with him. Now it's too late. I didn't want to make the same mistake with my mum, so I was going to call round to see her and make an effort, but I shan't bother now. Sod her.' Cheryl's tears had stopped and were replaced with contempt. She sat on her gran's sofa feeling tense. But when Bobby slipped his hand into hers, her shoulders relaxed and she looked sideways at him with a small smile. 'Thanks for coming with me today. I'm sorry that you saw my mum like that.'

Bobby gently squeezed her hand. 'I've met your family, so I think it's about time that you met mine.'

'Don't look so worried,' Edie piped up. 'I've known Bobby's family for years. They're smashing people and they'll love you.'

'Thanks, Edie. And your gran is right. My mum will love you.'

Cheryl hadn't considered meeting Bobby's family yet. But if he was ready to introduce her to them, then it meant he must be serious about their relationship. She felt a little flutter in her stomach. Bobby was *the one*, she was sure of that, but she wished he could have met her dad. And then a sad thought occurred to her – her father would never walk her down the aisle.

'Would you like to meet them tomorrow? Come for Sunday dinner. And you, Edie?'

'Don't you think you should check with your mum first?' Cheryl asked.

'No need. My mum has already been on at me about inviting you round. She'll be more than happy about you both coming for dinner tomorrow.'

'In that case, we'd love to,' Edie answered. 'I reckon we could both do with a bit of cheering up and your mum is always good company.'

Cheryl's mind was already racing about what she should wear to make a good impression. And should she take Bobby's mum a small gift? A gesture to say 'thank you'. Maybe some flowers? After all, though Cheryl hardly dared to think it, one day, Bobby's mum might become her mother-in-law.

27

Winnie rocked Martha in her arms and gazed lovingly at the baby. She could see David in her features but would never mention so to Rachel. Winnie's heart ached for her son. She'd never forgive him but she couldn't help worrying about him. She wondered if David had any idea that his father was dead. She doubted it.

'Has she fallen asleep?' Rachel asked.

'No, love. She's smiling at me.'

'Good, I haven't fed her yet.'

' 'Ere you are,' Winnie said, gently handing Martha back to Rachel. 'You see to her. I'd best get my pub open.'

'I'll be down as soon as she's settled.'

Winnie trudged down the stairs, aching all over. The nights in the cellar were taking its toll and she felt she could do with a day off from working. She loved her pub, even more so now that it was all hers. The Battersea Tavern was her pride and joy, a place where her customers were her friends. But feeling weary from sleepless nights, Winnie knew that today was going to be an effort to get through.

She'd only just opened when Hilda came through the door, her face ashen.

'That's not good for business,' Hilda said, indicating over her shoulder to the door.

'What's not?'

'Errol's outside and he's holding Bernie up against the wall.'

'He's what?'

'Threatening him, I reckon. I should have said something but Errol frightens the life out of me.'

'He don't scare me,' Winnie growled. She pulled up the sleeves of her cardigan and clomped across the pub. She meant business! How dare Errol intimidate her customers, especially Bernie, who'd never hurt a fly and was the size of a flea compared to Errol.

Winnie opened the door and stepped out onto the street. She saw Bernie cowering on the ground with Errol towering over him.

'Leave him alone!'

Errol didn't even look up. As Winnie marched towards him, Errol kicked Bernie, catching him in the ribs.

'*I said, leave him alone!*'

This time, Errol turned to her and Winnie was scared at what she saw. Errol's eyes were dark with rage and he was breathing heavily. She dashed to Bernie's side and crouched beside him. 'Come on, love, come inside and I'll get you cleaned up,' she soothed while glaring back at Errol.

'He asked for it,' Errol snarled. 'He owes me money.'

Winnie helped Bernie to his feet and urged him through the door. Then she turned and stood on the threshold with her hands on her hips. 'I don't care what he owes you. I warned you about this, Errol. I won't have this on my doorstep. In future, I suggest you conduct your business elsewhere.'

Errol stepped towards her until he was uncomfortably close. 'I'll conduct my business where I see fit,' he hissed.

'Not in my pub, you won't.'

'We'll see about that.'

Winnie shook her head in disgust at Errol and then went inside. Quickly she bolted the door. She looked around for Bernie and saw him sitting at a table with his head in his hands.

'It's all right, love, he won't be coming in. You're safe in here.'

Bernie shot her a fearful look. 'But I can't stay in here forever. He'll get me. One way or another,' he said, wincing in pain.

Winnie went behind the bar and poured a large brandy. 'This will help calm you down,' she told him. 'What on earth were you thinking? Getting into debt with Errol.'

'I weren't! I mean, I ain't in debt. I don't owe him a flamin' penny! He's stitched me up.'

'How?'

'I bought some eggs, cheese, ham and a few bits from him on tick last week. When I paid him today, he'd doubled the price with interest. It ain't on. Harry would be doing his nut. I always got stuff on tick from him but he never hiked the prices. Errol Hampton is a bleedin' disgrace to his father's name.'

Winnie shook her head. She'd been a fool to trust Errol. And now she feared she'd invited trouble to her door.

'Thanks, Winnie. I feel a bit better,' Bernie said. He placed the empty brandy glass on the table and then winced as he rose to his feet. 'I'd better get off. Cor, I can hardly get me breath, me ribs are killing me.'

'You're welcome to stay here for as long as you need.'

'No, I want to get home. Thanks. Wish me luck.'

'Take care, love. If you see him outside, make sure you come straight back here.'

'Will do. See ya.'

Winnie locked the door behind him and sighed. But then a knock on the door jolted her. She looked over at Hilda. 'I hope it's not Errol.'

'Shall I go out the back door and run to the phone box? I can call the police.'

'No. Errol is a bully. He feeds on fear. The best way to deal with him is to confront him.' She turned around, unbolted the door and threw it open, her face like thunder.

'Whoa, who's upset you?' Len asked as he stepped quickly backwards.

'Sorry, love. I thought you was Errol Hampton. Come in.'

After bolting the door again, Winnie served Len his bottle of stout in his pewter tankard.

'I take it Errol has been causing trouble again?'

'Yeah. He was outside earlier, giving Bernie a good hiding.'

'But Winnie stopped him,' Hilda added.

'What had Bernie done? He's harmless.'

'I know. But he'd bought some stuff from Errol last week on tick and then Errol doubled the price.'

'Cheeky git. He ain't going to be popular if that's how he's going to run his business. I've never bought a thing from him and never would.'

'Well, he won't be flogging his gear in here no more.'

'I'll go upstairs, if you're all right, Win?' Hilda asked.

'Yes, love. I'm fine.'

'Are you going to open up?'

'Of course. I won't let the likes of Errol get to me.' Winnie went to the door again and, though she was full of bravado, her nerves were jangled. Errol frightened her but she had to appear to be in control. She stepped into the street and looked up and down. There was no sign of him at the moment but Winnie knew that Errol would be back. And when he was, she'd have a battle on her hands.

Bobby came down the stairs from his bedroom to be greeted with the delicious aroma of his mum's Sunday roast cooking in the oven. He walked into the kitchen to find her spreading jam between two slabs of sponge cake. 'That looks nice.'

'I hope it tastes as nice as it looks,' she answered. Then she glanced up from the cake and eyed him up and down. 'Well, well, well. You look very nice yourself,' she said with a broad smile. 'You've certainly made an effort.'

'Thanks, Mum. It's not too much, is it?'

'No, not at all. I've always liked that suit on you. Though you're going to make me and your father look like a right pair of scruffbags.'

'Don't talk soft. Talking of Dad, where is he?'

'Down the pub. But don't worry, he knows he's got to be home in good time and I've told him he wasn't to have more than two halves. You know what a silly beggar he becomes if he has any more than that. I wouldn't want him showing us up.'

After Cheryl's mum's performance in the pub yesterday, Bobby thought his father would have to go a long way to show them up! Anyway, his dad was never horrible when drunk. Just a bit of a clown – and loud.

'Are you sure they're both up to visiting today? I don't think I'd be in any fit state to be calling in to friends and neighbours if anything happened to you or your father.'

'They're fine, Mum. I mean, they're coping well.'

'Edie's always been a strong woman. Don't let that little-old-lady-act fool you. She's as strong as an ox and brave too. Years ago, when, you was in your pram, I was out shopping and I bumped into Edie. We were having a chat outside the jeweller's when, all of a sudden, this bloke ran out of the shop and fell over your pram. The shopkeeper rushed out, shouting "Thief!". Well, as the bloke was scrambling back to his feet, Edie, as quick as a streak of lightening, jumped on him and held him down on the ground. She got an award from the police and was in the local paper.'

Bobby grinned at the image of Edie wrestling with a jewel thief. 'Oh, Mum, you must tell Cheryl about that.'

'I've got plenty more stories like that about Edie. She was quite the celebrity in Balham. After her son Wilf was killed in France, Edie went to work for the London Omnibus Company. Women weren't paid nearly as much as men and the unions didn't like having women in the work force. Edie stood up to them. She was one of the founding members of an all-women union. And she fought hard for women's rights, even protesting outside Wandsworth Town Hall.'

'Well, I'll be buggered.'

'Oi, language. I hope you don't swear like that in front of Edie!'

'Sorry, Mum. I'm just surprised to hear all that about Edie.'

'If Cheryl is anything like her grandmother, you'll have a good woman.'

Bobby recalled the day before when Edie had whacked Cheryl's mother across the face. Edie was a pint-sized woman, just like Cheryl, but clearly a formidable force to be reckoned with. Bobby liked that. And though he hadn't seen it yet, he was sure that Cheryl had that same fortitude.

They heard the front door open and his dad called, 'Alice, look who I found on me way home.'

Bobby walked into the passageway to see his dad ushering Cheryl and Edie in with him. 'Hello. You've met my dad, then,' he said to Cheryl. 'Let me take your coats.'

Bobby helped Edie off with hers and placed both coats over the bannisters. 'Come through, it's a lot warmer in the front room.'

Cheryl looked nervous but Bobby knew that his mum would soon put her at ease. He invited them to sit on the sofa and then his mum came into the room.

'I'm so pleased you could come today,' she gushed. 'I'm Alice. Bobby's told me lots about you. You're working in Barratt's? That's wonderful, I love their shoes. Are you set-tling in well in Balham? It's a lot smaller and quieter than Battersea.'

'Mum, give Cheryl a chance; she's only just walked through the door.'

'Sorry. Would you like a cup of tea or a cold drink?'

'I'd love a cup of tea, thank you.'

'Me an' all. I thought you was never going to ask,' Edie said and chuckled.

'Can I give you a hand?' Cheryl offered.

'No, thank you. But Bobby and his father can pull the table out. Where is your dad?' she asked Bobby.

'In the privy.'

'Right, let me get you that tea. Bobby, put some more coal on the fire.'

A couple of hours later, they sat around the table, finishing their dinner. Bobby was pleased to see that his mum and Cheryl were getting along. His mum had filled the conversation with her stories about Edie, which Cheryl had relished. And though Edie had appeared embarrassed at first, it was clear that she was proud of her past achievements.

'That was a smashing roast, thank you. And thank you for entertaining me,' Cheryl said. 'I had no idea my gran was such a little firecracker.'

'You're more than welcome. Come round whenever you like. There's loads more I can tell you about Edie.'

'Yes, thanks, Alice, today has been just the ticket. We needed this after the week we've had,' Edie said.

Bobby reached beside him and placed his hand on top of Cheryl's. She was puffy around the eyes from the tears that she'd cried yesterday but he thought she still looked stunning. He'd have liked to have taken her up to his room and been alone with her but he knew his mother would never allow it. This evening, however, if they had the inevitable attack from the German bombers, Bobby planned to shelter on the underground platform with Cheryl instead of in the Anderson in their back garden.

He looked down the table at his father. His dad gave him an approving look. Cheryl had won the hearts of his parents, just as she'd won his.

28

Rachel came into the front room carrying Martha who was gurgling happily. 'Are we disturbing you?' she asked.

Winnie had been listening to the wireless but there was nothing of any interest to her that was being broadcast. 'No, love. It's all talk about Churchill being elected head of the Conservative party.'

'I've never taken much notice of politics but a lot of people are saying that Mr Churchill will lead the country to victory.'

'I hope he does it quickly. I don't know how much longer I can stand being stuck down in the cellar.'

'I know what you mean. But at least Martha doesn't seem to mind it. Thank goodness she's got used to the sound of Moaning Minnie too. The poor mite used to scream her head off but she takes it all in her stride now.'

'I know, bless her, but it ain't right. All them poor kiddies sent out of London and away from their parents. Mind you, at least they're getting some healthy country air and not breathing in the muck round here. I suppose I should go and open up. Switch the wireless off when you come down.'

The morning ticked by with a steady flow of customers.

Some spoke about Chamberlain retiring completely from politics and Churchill succeeding him as party leader. Others, like Winnie, didn't have much to say about it.

'You might as well go back upstairs, love,' Winnie told Rachel. 'I'm not rushed off my feet today.'

'Are you sure?'

'Yeah, go and put your feet up. You can do our supper tonight, how's that for a deal?'

'Deal,' Rachel chirped. 'Give me a shout if you need me.'

Winnie looked around her pub and smiled to herself. She reckoned the war would be over before some of her customers finished their drinks. Cor, talk about nursing an ale! But then, she supposed, there was no rush. Her relaxed mood changed instantly when Errol walked in.

It had been five days since she'd warned him that he was no longer welcome in her pub. Winnie tensed as Errol sauntered towards the bar as if he didn't have a care in the world. Her customers fell quiet. She could feel the jittery atmosphere. No one had been happy about Errol's actions though Winnie thought that there were few who'd be willing to challenge him. She had a pub full of men, mostly elderly, but she felt very alone.

'What do you want?' she asked him sternly.

'A drink. This is still a pub, ain't it?'

'Yes, but not one that you'll be drinking in. Bernie has two cracked ribs, thanks to you.'

'Hmm, maybe I was a bit hard on him. But me and Bernie are all square now. I let him off the hook.'

'I don't care, Errol. I don't like the way you operate and I won't have my customers conned or beaten. So you can sling your hook and take your custom elsewhere. There's no one in my pub who wants to buy anything from you.'

Errol looked down at his shining shoes and when he raised his face again, Winnie recognised his dark expression. It was the one she'd seen after he'd kicked Bernie. He glared at her in the same way Brian used to before he'd thump her. Winnie nervously licked her dry lips. She quickly reminded herself that she'd stood up to Brian and she could do the same with Errol.

Errol fished in his pocket and then slammed a few coins on the counter. It soon became clear to Winnie that he had no intention of going quietly. *Thank goodness Rachel is upstairs,* she thought, grateful that the girl wouldn't be involved.

'My usual,' Errol ordered.

'Take your money and go. I won't serve you so you're wasting your time.'

Without saying a word, Errol stomped along the bar. To Winnie's horror, he lifted the hatch and was now on the same side of the counter as her. Without the bar between them, she suddenly felt very vulnerable.

'Oi, what do you think you're doing?' Len called.

'I'm getting meself a drink, old man.'

'You can't do that.'

Errol thudded towards Len. He leaned across the bar and sneered. 'I can do whatever I want, so button it.'

Len climbed down from his stool and clenched his fists. 'Outside,' he barked.

Errol threw his head back and laughed. 'Are you challenging me? Sit down, you soppy old git.'

'I was a champion boxer in me day. I ain't scared of a

scallywag like you. Come on, outside. I'll show you. I'll put you on your arse where you belong.'

'Len, please, leave it,' Winnie begged.

'Yeah, old man. Leave it,' Errol repeated.

Another two old fellas edged towards the bar. They were soon followed by four elderly chaps who'd been sitting in the corner playing cards. Winnie looked on astonished. She couldn't believe that her old and loyal customers were coming forward to protect her and Len.

'Ha, what's this?' Errol said, smirking. 'What do you think you lot are going to do? Whack me with your walking sticks? Oooo, I'm scared,' he mocked.

'Get out, Son, or we'll make you sorry,' Len warned.

'You heard him,' Winnie said bravely. 'Don't push your luck.'

Errol, laughing derisively, turned and grabbed a glass tumbler which he then began to fill with whisky.

Winnie walked towards him and whispered, 'You'll achieve nothing in here by trying to be the big man. My lot can see straight through you. You're a sad man, Errol. We ain't impressed and you don't scare us. Just go, eh?' she said. 'Save us all a load of bother.'

Errol knocked back his drink and banged his empty glass on the counter. His eyes fixed on the wall mirror behind the bar. Winnie was standing beside him and she reached for his empty glass, hoping that he'd leave now. As she went to pick up the glass, Errol's arm swung out. The back of his fist pounded against the side of her head, sending her reeling.

Stunned, her head throbbing, Winnie looked up from the floor. Errol stood over her. He appeared to be shocked. 'Sorry ... I-I-I didn't mean ...' he stuttered. He reached down, offering a hand, but Winnie recoiled. The next thing she knew, four or five of the old blokes, including Len, were all over Errol.

'You bastard,' Len hissed as he tugged on Errol's arm. Between them, they pulled Errol from behind the bar.

Winnie rose to her feet, shakily, and looked over the bar to see them taking Errol towards the door. He offered no resistance and was mumbling how sorry he was and that he hadn't meant to lash out. Winnie had no sympathy for him. She'd had enough of men beating her!

As the door closed behind him, dazed and confused, she rubbed her sore head. 'How did that happen?' she mumbled.

Len was beside her now. 'Come and sit down, pet.'

He led her to a table and someone handed her a glass of brandy.

'What's wrong with Winnie?' Rachel asked.

Winnie looked up and saw the girl behind the bar. 'I'm all right, love. I just had a bit of a run-in with Errol. But he didn't give me any worse than my husband used to. And thanks to this lot, he's gone.'

Rachel ran from behind the bar and dropped by Winnie's side. 'Did he hit you?'

'Yeah, but I'm fine.'

'I'm calling the police. He's not getting away with this.'

'There's no need. It's done and dusted now.'

'There's every need. What if he comes back and does it again? No, Win, he needs locking up!'

'She's right,' Len said. 'He should be behind bars. And you've got a pub full of witnesses who'll be willing to testify.'

Winnie realised that they were talking sense. Errol shouldn't be allowed to walk around punching women, or anyone else for that matter! 'Go and call them,' she told Rachel.

As Winnie sat with her customers fussing over her, she thought about how different things were when Harry had been around. He'd be so ashamed of Errol. The poor man would be turning in his grave. But as Winnie began to think more clearly, though she felt awful for doing it, she was determined to send down Harry's son. And Battersea would be a better place without him.

29

Cheryl was glad to have finished work on Saturday. Her new shoes had given her raw blisters on the backs of her heels. It felt such a relief to kick the shoes off her sore feet.

She glanced at the clock. Errol and Yvonne were late. Cheryl hoped that Yvonne would arrive soon or they'd be keeping Bobby and Ken waiting. Though she supposed that it didn't really matter if they were late, as their date consisted of a few card games and a singalong on the crammed platform of Balham underground station. Still, they had to make the best of things and at least they were together down there, and safe.

At last, there was a knock on the front door. 'That'll be Errol and Yvonne,' Edie said, smiling widely. Cheryl's gran always seemed to be over the moon at seeing Errol. And funnily enough, Errol enjoyed the old girl's company too. Cheryl had been pleasantly surprised at how well the pair got along. It warmed her heart and she thought it was a joy to see.

Cheryl opened the door and looked over Yvonne's shoulder. 'Hello. Where's me brother?' she asked.

'I got the bus over.'

'Oh, I thought Errol was bringing you here. Come in. My gran will be disappointed that he isn't with you.'

In the front room, Yvonne sat on the cane chair but appeared to be fidgeting nervously. Cheryl sensed that something was wrong and braced herself for more bad news, though nothing could be as horrific as when she'd been told of her dad's death. But where was Errol? Fear flooded through her as it occurred to her that he might have been killed too. 'Out with it,' she demanded.

Yvonne pursed her lips but before she could speak, Edie cried, 'Please, no, not Errol? I can't lose him too.'

'No, Errol's not dead,' Yvonne blurted with urgency. 'But he's been arrested.'

'What?' Cheryl spat. 'Why?'

'Apparently, he attacked Mrs Berry. Punched her and knocked her to the floor. Then when the police went to arrest him, he had a fight with them an' all. I heard it took four coppers to hold him down.'

'Oh my goodness!' Edie said in disbelief.

Cheryl felt the blood drain from her face. 'He hit Mrs Berry? Why? Why would he do that? My brother can be a beast but I've never known him to hit a woman!'

'I don't know why he did it. I think she tried to throw him out of the pub.'

'I can't believe it. And fighting coppers. He'll do time for that!'

'That's what everyone is saying. No one thinks that he'll be out for a while.'

'I'm sorry. I know he's my grandson but there's no excuse

for him hitting Mrs Berry. If it's true and that's what he did, then he deserves to go to prison.'

'But, Gran—'

'But nothing. It'll teach him a lesson. He'll think twice before he raises his fists to a woman again. A short, sharp shock. It'll do him good.'

'Do you really believe that, Gran?'

'Yes, dear, I do. I don't like to think of him locked away behind bars but he'll do his time and then we'll be here for him when he gets out.'

Cheryl wasn't so sure. It broke her heart to think of her brother in prison and enduring the harsh regime. And what about their mum? Errol had been taking care of her. Cheryl couldn't afford to pay her mother's rent. But she'd worry about that later. Right now, she was more concerned about her brother. 'What do we do? Can we visit him? Take him some things he might need?'

Eddie shook her head. 'I don't know. I've never known anyone who's been arrested. I should imagine that he's in a police cell and I doubt that anyone will be permitted to see him. Oh, the silly boy.'

'Honestly, Gran, it's just one thing on top of another. How much more bad luck can my family take?'

'This ain't bad luck. This is down to your brother's complete stupidity.'

'How's Mrs Berry, do you know?' Cheryl asked Yvonne.

'I think she's all right. The pub is open but I've not been in.'

Cheryl thought for a moment. 'I think we should go and see her and apologise.'

Edie leaned forward in her chair. 'I'm not apologising for

324

Errol's actions. Your brother is the one who needs to say sorry to her, not us. We ain't done nothing wrong!'

'I can't think straight. My mind is working overtime. It's not sunk in that my brother is going to prison!'

'Put the kettle on. Let's have a cup of tea. And you may as well fill your face with them biscuits I made for Errol. He won't be having them now.'

No, he won't, thought Cheryl. Errol wouldn't be enjoying any home comforts for a good while to come. She had no idea when she'd see him again, and right now, more than ever, she needed her brother. After her father's death, Errol had promised to look after her, but now, due to his despicable and inexplicable actions, she'd been left alone. And so had their mum. *Thanks,* she thought, *thanks a flamin' lot!*

A tender lump had formed on the side of Winnie's head but she was glad that the headache had passed. She'd heard about Errol's arrest and how he'd struck two of the policemen. That was bound to guarantee his incarceration and Winnie thought good riddance to him. But she wondered, with Harry dead and Errol locked up, who would take over selling the black-market goods. After all, it had shown itself to be a lucrative business, one from which she had profited too. And though it was illegal, she'd miss her extras to top up her rations.

'How's your head?' Rachel asked.

'Sore. I was just thinking about Errol's business. I suppose someone else will step into his shoes.'

'Yes, probably.'

'I wonder who Errol and Harry bought the stuff from. Have you got any idea?'

'No, not a clue, Win.'

'Hmm, that's a shame. Perhaps if we ask around, we could find out.'

'Why do we want to know? Oh, hang on … please tell me that you're not thinking of buying and flogging black-market stuff?'

'Well, if someone's going to make a profit from it, why not us?'

'No, Win, I don't want any part of it! I'm a mother. I've got Martha to think about.'

Winnie was quiet for a moment and then she laughed. 'You silly moo, I'm only joking. I don't mind buying a bit here and there, especially eggs and cheese, but I couldn't be a spiv. Your face was a picture though.'

'You had me going for a minute then. I thought that whack to your head had sent you doolally.'

'Nope, I've still got all my facilities – well, most of 'em. But I have been doing some thinking and we really do need an extra pair of hands around here.'

'Yes, I think you're right. I'm just so nervous after what happened with Lucy.'

'That's understandable, love. I rushed into offering Lucy a job and a home but I knew very little about the girl, God rest her soul. But we'll be extra careful this time.'

Winnie had been thinking hard about who she could offer the position to. Food, petrol and other household basics weren't the only shortages. There was a lack of available working women as well. Many had joined the war effort; they'd either been drafted or had volunteered. And there was absolutely no way that Winnie would employ a man, not if he were to live on the premises too. It was bad enough that Rachel's reputation was already tarnished and that her child was brandished a bastard. Winnie wouldn't feed the gossipmongers by giving them something else to talk about. And a young man living under their roof would certainly get the tongues wagging. Anyway, she'd feel much more relaxed in the company of a woman and she knew that Rachel would too.

A man came in whom Winnie didn't recognise. A young bloke, smartly dressed, rather unassuming. Rachel was quick to serve him and when she'd finished, Winnie asked, 'Who's that?'

'No idea.'

Winnie served a customer but she was aware of the stranger's eyes following her. Every time that she sneaked a peek at him, he was quick to look the other way. Once he'd finished his drink, he signed for another. Winnie told Rachel that she'd see to him.

'Same again?' she asked.

'Yes, please.'

Winnie placed his drink on the bar and took his money.

'Keep the change.'

She threw the coins in the tip glass and wandered back over to him. 'What brings you in here?'

'Nothing much. I was in the area. Is this where the punch-up happened with Errol and the landlady?'

'Who are you?' she asked suspiciously.

'No one special. Are you the landlady?'

'I am.'

'Mrs Winnie Berry?'

'That's my name, don't wear it out.'

'What happened, then? Was Errol drunk and you threw him out?'

'Something like that.'

'Is it true that he was selling black-market goods in here?'

'What are you, a copper?'

'No, Mrs Berry.'

'Well, I don't like your questioning, young man. So finish your drink in quiet or change the subject.'

'Sorry. Look, I'll be honest with you. I'm a reporter from the local paper. We're running the story about Errol Hampton's arrest and I'd like to get your perspective on it.'

'Get stuffed! I don't want my name in the papers and certainly not associated with Errol Hampton.'

'The paper is going to print the story so you might as well get your side across.'

'No, thank you. Print what you like but you won't get a story or a quote from me.'

'Please, Mrs Berry. Give me a break. I'm new in the job and an interview with you will impress my editor.'

Winnie thought for a moment. 'You can print this,' she said. 'Errol Hampton punched me to the ground after I refused to serve him and wouldn't permit him to trade in black-market stock in my pub. There, that's all you're getting.'

'I was told this was a hub for getting my hands on anything I wanted. Wasn't Errol's father, Harry Hampton, selling from here too?'

'No, he wasn't. He'd pop in sometimes for a drink but he knew the rules and respected them. If there was any illegal trading going on, then it was happening outside of my door.'

The reporter scribbled a few notes in a small notepad. 'Just one more thing, Mrs Berry. Your son, David Berry. What was his involvement in the kidnapping of your granddaughter and the suicide of Lucy Little?'

'That's enough! Take your rag and your gossip out of my pub. I shan't have my name dragged through the mud for the entertainment of your readers or to help you get promoted. Go on, bugger off and don't come back!'

The reporter threw the rest of his drink down his neck. 'Thanks, Mrs Berry. It was nice meeting you and you've been very helpful.'

Winnie's stomach knotted as she watched him walk out.

'What was all that about?' Rachel asked.

'He was a reporter and was asking questions about Errol and Harry. Then he brought up David and Lucy. I'm afraid they're going to run a story about me and all of us. I don't think it will be pretty reading.'

'What did you tell him?'

'Nothing, I hope. But he was asking about the black market. I denied that any selling went on in here. But I don't think he believed me.'

'They can't prove anything. You've got nothing to worry about.'

'I hope not, I really hope not,' Winnie said. She dreaded to think what the paper was going to say about her, her family and her pub. But whatever it was, Winnie suspected that they weren't going to be shown in a good light. She'd soon find out. The paper would be for sale on Tuesday. She had three days to worry about it and then all of the borough would know her business.

30

The following day, Cheryl and Bobby arrived back at her gran's, both stuffed with Bobby's mum's Sunday roast. Edie hadn't wanted to join them, saying that she was tired and was going to enjoy an afternoon nap. Cheryl hoped that her gran was awake now and that they weren't disturbing her.

'Shush, keep your voice down in case me gran is still sleeping,' she whispered.

'I can hear you,' Edie called. 'And I'm wide awake.'

Cheryl exchanged a smile with Bobby. When they went into the front room, Edie was sitting in her chair but she'd pulled it closer to the sideboard.

'What are you doing over there?' Cheryl asked.

'Look, it says here in my *Radio Times* that Princess Elizabeth is going to address the children of the commonwealth. She's only fourteen, bless her cotton socks. Such a wise head on her little young shoulders. She's going to do a broadcast with Uncle Mac on *Children's Hour*. I'm sitting over here so that I can hear the wireless better.'

'You want to listen to *Children's Hour*?'

'Not normally, no. But I'd like to hear the princess. So, if you two can't keep quiet for an hour, then I suggest you go for a walk or something.'

'Do you want to listen to the princess?' Cheryl asked Bobby.

'Not really. But I will if you do.'

'No, come on. Let's leave me gran to it. We'll be back in an hour, Gran.'

'All right, dear. Keep warm.'

'Don't worry, I'll keep you warm,' Bobby whispered.

'I heard that an' all,' Edie said. 'Me eyesight might be going but there's nothing wrong with my hearing. You keep your mucky paws off my granddaughter or you'll have me to answer to.'

Again, Cheryl and Bobby exchanged a smile.

Outside, it was dry but chilly. Cheryl looped her arm through Bobby's. 'I wonder if Yvonne and Ken enjoyed their afternoon without us.'

'I should think so. Ken is pretty keen on Yvonne. How does she feel about him?'

'I'm not telling you so that you can go running off to Ken and tell him. Some things should remain a mystery and the fella has to find out for himself.'

'Oh, go on, Cheryl. Give me a clue, at least.'

'What's it worth?' Cheryl teased.

'Four chicken drumsticks?'

'You'll have to do better than that!'

'What about this, then?' Bobby said. He pulled a small box from his coat pocket and dropped to one knee.

'What are you doing?'

Bobby opened the box to reveal a gold ring with a row

of three small diamonds across it. He smiled nervously and then asked, 'Will you marry me?'

Cheryl gasped and both her hands flew over her mouth. She stared down at Bobby, her mind turning. She'd dreamed of marrying him, but not yet. They'd only known each other for a few weeks.

Bobby seemed to sense her hesitancy and asked, 'If you can't say yes now, will you at least think about it?'

'Yes.'

'Yes, you'll marry me or yes, you'll think about it?'

'I'll think about it.'

Bobby stood up and kissed Cheryl's cheek. 'That's all I ask. I realise it's a bit of a surprise to you but I know that you're the girl for me.'

'I think the world of you, I really do, Bobby. It's just so soon.'

'I know. But lots of sweethearts are marrying quickly.'

'Yeah, because the fellas are going off to fight. But you're here with me. We get to spend most nights together.'

'You, me, your gran and about six hundred more people. Not to mention the passengers getting on and off the trains,' Bobby replied with a chuckle.

'But my point is, we're together. We don't need to rush into anything.'

'The thing is ... I won't be seeing quite so much of you.'

'Why not?'

'I've joined the Home Guard. I'll be away a fair bit doing training.'

'The Home Guard?'

'Yes. The army wouldn't have me so I've signed up with the volunteers.'

'That's a very worthy thing to do. I'm proud of you.'

'Proud enough to marry me?' Bobby asked cheekily.

'We'll see. That's as much as I can promise for now. Your proposal has come right out of the blue and on top of everything else that's happened lately – I'm sort of reeling a bit.'

'I'm sorry. I should have waited, especially after your dad and your brother. This is probably the last thing you need but I reasoned with myself that it might help to take your mind off things.'

Cheryl stood on her tiptoes and placed a long and gentle kiss on Bobby's lips. 'I'm flattered that you've asked me to be your wife and I haven't said no. It's just a bit of a surprise. A nice one, mind.'

'Just don't leave me on tenterhooks for too long, eh?'

'I won't, I promise. I need a day or two to get my head around it and mull it over. But as soon as I've made up my mind, you'll be the first to know.'

'If you decide you're not ready yet, that doesn't mean it's the end of us. I'll wait, however long it takes. You'll be my wife one day.'

Cheryl gazed deeply into Bobby's eyes. It would be so easy to say yes to him. But she'd always credited herself with being sensible and rushing into marrying a man she barely knew would be a reckless thing to do. Her head ruled her heart but her heart was telling her to say yes.

Bobby changed the subject back to their friends. 'So, what about Yvonne? Is she keen on Ken?'

'Yeah, I think so. She's had a crush on Errol for years but now all she talks about is Ken. Why do you ask? Is he thinking of proposing too?'

'Christ, no. Ken's not as mad as me. He warned me not to ask you. He said it was too soon.'

'Sensible man. He'll be surprised if I say yes.'

'Not as surprised as I will be,' Bobby said lightly.

They passed the tube station, both noticing that a queue was already beginning to form. 'I think we should head back now and get Gran.'

'Are you going to tell her?'

'What, that you've proposed to me? No, of course I'm not. I won't hear the last of it. She'll be in my ear all night telling me to say yes. She thinks you're the best thing since sliced bread.'

'I might tell her, then,' Bobby joked.

Cheryl had already decided that she wouldn't mention Bobby's proposal to her gran. Edie wouldn't offer her an objective opinion. But her mum would. Cheryl had an over-whelming urge to talk to her. They'd never been close but her mother had always offered good advice. And right now, that's what Cheryl felt she needed. But her mother had hurt Cheryl deeply and angered her. Still, she'd found herself softening and she worried how her mother was coping financially without Errol to help. Cheryl decided that she'd visit her mother as soon as she could. And only after that would she give Bobby his answer.

As they strolled back up the hill, although she felt elated at Bobby's proposal, she couldn't shake the tinge of sadness that marred it. She had no dad to walk her down the aisle and now neither could her older brother.

'You're thinking about it, aren't you?' Bobby asked.

'I said I would,' she answered, forcing a smile.

As if reading her mind, Bobby said, 'I'm sorry about my

timing. You're still in shock about your dad and now your brother. I know that if you agree to be my wife, you'll miss them both on our wedding day.'

Tears pricked Cheryl's eyes. Bobby was so sensitive and thoughtful. She felt silly for trying to hide her pain from him. 'I've no one to walk me down the aisle,' she cried.

'Your dad will always be with you. I hope he approves of me.'

'He'd love you,' Cheryl sniffed. 'Just like I do.'

She felt her feet almost lift from the ground as Bobby scooped her up into his arms. 'I love you too,' he said huskily in her ear.

Cheryl felt safe there and wished that they could stay in that moment forever. She'd told him that she loved him. She was sure that she did. But was she sure enough to commit to spending the rest of her life with him? That would take some thought and now, more than ever, she knew she had to talk to her mum.

Winnie poured Bill and his wife, Flo, a drink. 'On me,' she said quietly.

'Cheers, Winnie.'

'We don't often get the pleasure of your company on a Sunday afternoon. Are you celebrating?'

'No, I wish we were,' Bill answered.

And Flo added, 'My niece, her husband and their five kids are staying at ours. They got bombed out, we had no choice but to offer them a home. So now we're living on top of each other and I'm not used to the noise levels. Why do children sound so whiny?'

'Gawd knows. If they aren't whining then they're screeching. It's good of you to put them up.'

'I hope it won't be for too long. Don't get me wrong, they're a smashing family but our Anderson only has room for six people. It's crammed enough with just me and Bill. It's near on impossible with my niece and the rest of them. We shall have to use the public shelter tonight but I'm not looking forward to that,' Flo moaned, wrinkling her nose.

'We can't have that. You and Bill can stay here tonight, down in my cellar. It's just as good as any public shelter but a darn sight more comfortable.'

'Oh, no, Winnie, I wasn't dropping hints!'

'I know you weren't. But I insist. I've got spare bedding down there, lights, grub and drinks. If there's any home comforts you want with you, go and collect them now.'

'Are you sure?' Bill asked.

'I said so, didn't I? Me and Rachel will be glad of the company.'

'Doesn't Hilda use your cellar?' Flo asked.

'No,' Winnie answered. She hid a wry smile. Hilda and Bill had always rubbed along together nicely, much to Flo's annoyance. In fact, Bill had been one of the few people who'd had the patience to tolerate Hilda when she'd been drunk. Winnie was sure that Hilda had a soft spot for Bill and thought that he most likely had one for Hilda too.

'Well, thank you very much, Winnie. We'd love to accept your generous invitation. I can't say that I was looking forward to spending a night in the public shelter. I'll pop home and get my knitting. Shall I grab your book, Bill?'

'Yes, and don't forget my spectacles.'

Later that evening, once the pub had closed, Bill helped

Winnie to clean and tidy up. Flo returned and mucked in too. Winnie enjoyed their company and the light-hearted chat. It kept her mind off worrying about the dreaded newspaper article that was going to be run on Tuesday. But their cheerful conversation was interrupted by the sound of the all-too-familiar air-raid siren.

'Here we go again,' Bill moaned.

'They're early today,' Flo said, looking at the wall clock behind the bar.

'Right, let's go downstairs and get settled in for the night,' Winnie said. She led the way down to the cellar with Rachel and Martha following too.

'It's smashing down here,' Flo said in awe as she glanced around.

'Thanks. We've tried to make it as comfortable as possible. Make yourself at home. There's a bucket behind those barrels over there. It's not the most ideal privy but it's private enough and we have to make do.'

'It's fine, thank you,' Flo said. 'It's much better than our Anderson. To be honest, Winnie, there's been nights when I've thought about staying in my bed and taking my chances with the bombs. I hate that Anderson. It's a miserable place; cold, damp and smelly. Not to mention the spiders and bugs. Your cellar is luxury in comparison.'

Winnie felt proud of herself for creating a homely space for them to shelter in. She thought that she and Rachel were luckier than most. She hadn't been inside an Anderson but had heard plenty of her customers moan about them. They didn't sound like nice places to have to spend the night. 'You and Bill are welcome to stay here whenever you like.'

As they made themselves comfortable and Winnie poured

them a ginger beer, the sound of muffled explosions reached their ears.

'They're close,' Bill said gravely.

Winnie shuddered and silently prayed that the Germans' bombs wouldn't come any closer. Martha began to cry in Rachel's arms. Winnie thought that her granddaughter had probably sensed Rachel's tension. 'Give her here,' she offered. 'Let her nanna have a cuddle.'

Rachel looked grateful as she passed her baby to Winnie. 'Thanks,' she whispered.

'Leave her with me. Try and get some rest. I'll wake you if she needs a feed.'

'She's a bonnie girl,' Flo cooed.

'She is but she's got a pair of lungs on her that could give Moaning Minnie a run for her money,' Winnie chuckled. 'There, there, there,' she soothed as she gently rocked Martha from side to side. 'We won't get much sleep unless Martha does.'

'I hope Bill's snoring doesn't disturb you,' Flo said quietly.

'It won't disturb me. I hardly sleep anyway and Rachel is a heavy sleeper, she can sleep through most things.' *Even someone sneaking into her bedroom to steal her child,* Winnie thought sadly.

A couple of hours later, Winnie looked over into the drawer beside her. Martha was sound asleep in the makeshift cot. Rachel was buried under a pile of blankets and Bill was snoring softly. She hadn't heard any explosions in a while but she knew it wasn't safe to venture from the cellar until they heard the all-clear.

'Are you awake?' Flo whispered.

'Yes, love. Are you?'

'No, I'm sleeping,' Flo giggled.

Winnie laughed quietly too. 'Silly moo.'

'There's something that's been playing on my mind. Bill said that I shouldn't say anything to you but I think you should know.'

'What?' Winnie asked.

'It's about Hilda.'

'What about her?'

'I saw her the other day. She was coming out of a pub on Falcon Road. Oh, Winnie, it was awful. She was staggering all over the place and gave me a right mouthful.'

'You're kidding me?'

'No, I wish I was. I thought she'd stopped drinking.'

'So did I! You're sure it was her?'

'Yes, it was her. She was a disgrace, swearing like an old fisherwoman. I left her to it.'

'Please don't say anything to Rachel about this.'

'No, of course I won't. It's horrible to see Hilda in that sort of mess.'

'I know. She's vile when she's drunk. Leave it with me, Flo. I'll have a word with her.'

'Good luck with that. I hope for Rachel's sake that you can make Hilda see sense.'

Winnie's lips pursed as she thought about drunken Hilda. The woman had caused no end of trouble and grief when she'd been fuelled by booze. And if Hilda was slipping back into her old ways, it would break Rachel's heart. This wouldn't do. They couldn't go back to dealing with Hilda in that state. Winnie would have to confront her and she would, as soon as morning broke and it was safe to go outside.

31

The following morning, Winnie was up early and dressed, ready to have it out with Hilda. She tiptoed through to the kitchen, surprised to find Bill and Flo also up and dressed.

'Good morning. Couldn't you get any sleep on the sofa, Bill?'

'Morning, Winnie. The sofa was very comfy, thanks, but me and Flo always have an early start for work.'

'Of course you do. The market doesn't set itself up. Were you all right in the little room, Flo?'

'It was perfect, thank you. It was quite nice to get away from Bill's snoring for a few hours. We didn't wake you, did we?'

'No, I'm off to see Hilda,' Winnie replied. She gave Flo a knowing look.

'There's tea in the pot, Winnie. Me and Flo can't thank you enough for last night.'

'I told you, you're welcome anytime. I suggest that all the while your niece and her family are at yours, you should stay here every night.'

'If you don't mind, Winnie, we'd love to take you up on that offer, thank you.'

'It's not a problem.'

'We'd better get to work. See you later.'

'Yes, see you.'

Winnie poured herself a cup of tea and drank it quickly. As she rinsed her cup and saucer in the sink, Rachel padded into the room. 'Morning, Win. You off out somewhere?'

'Hello, love, yes. I'm popping up the junction and want to get in the bread queue nice and early. I'll be back in time to open up.' She felt awful about telling fibs to Rachel, but, thankfully, the girl didn't question her any further. 'I'll see you soon, love,' Winnie said and she left the kitchen before Rachel could ask her anything.

The street was quiet but Winnie noticed a singed smell in the air, no doubt from the German bombardment last night. She shook her head and pushed all thoughts of the devastation around her from her mind. As she turned the corner, a strong gust of cold wind whipped up her coat. She tightened the knot of her headscarf under her chin and hoped this winter wouldn't be a harsh one. After all, the only heating they had in the pub and flat was from the chimneys and it was already a tedious chore to buy coal. The queues were horrendous and were only going to get worse. This blasted war, she thought. And to top it all, she'd have to start thinking about Christmas soon. Though Gawd knows what sort of festivities they'd have this year. But Winnie would make the most of what she could and would throw her traditional Christmas lunch. Maybe Hitler would give them a break for Christmas, but she doubted it.

Winnie was soon outside the house that Hilda shared. She

took a deep breath before marching to the front door and knocking hard on Hilda's window. When Hilda pulled back the curtains, Winnie's heart sank at the sight of the woman. Hilda's peroxide blonde, dishevelled hair and wrinkled clothes along with her pasty-looking skin and bleary eyes confirmed Winnie's fears. Hilda had obviously been drinking heavily again.

'Go away,' Hilda mouthed.

'No. Let me in.'

Hilda dropped the curtain and moments later, she pulled open the front door. Her head hung low and she slumped against the door frame.

'It's true, then. You're back on the booze.'

'I don't need a lecture from you.'

'Yes you do, Hilda Duff! You're going to listen to me even if I have to keep on at you until I'm blue in the face. Now, let me in and get the kettle on.'

'I haven't got any milk.'

'I'll take my tea black. Move.'

Hilda stepped aside and Winnie went in and through to Hilda's room. She was shocked at the state of it. Dirty clothes were strewn all over the floor. The overflowing ashtray had been knocked over and the place stank of foul body odour.

'This is disgusting,' Winnie spat.

'Yeah, well, you weren't invited. If you don't like it, feel free to bugger off.'

Winnie spun around and glared at Hilda. 'Why, Hilda? Why have you let yourself down?'

'I'll put the kettle on,' Hilda answered meekly.

While Hilda was in the kitchen, Winnie dashed about picking up clothes and tidying up. She threw the curtains wide open. The room had begun to resemble something like normal when Hilda returned with two cups.

'Thanks. My head is throbbing. I couldn't be bothered to clean up.'

'Your head is throbbing because you've been drinking.'

'Thanks for stating the obvious.'

They sat at Hilda's small drop-leaf table in front of the window. Hilda squinted her eyes and turned away from the low morning sunlight streaming through.

'Why have you messed up, Hilda? You were doing so well. Or has this been going on for a while?'

Hilda shook her head. 'It's been creeping up. It started with me just having a glass or two of whisky to calm my nerves. These bombs, Win, they terrify me. I've been a nervous wreck.'

'Oh, Hilda, you know what a glass or two leads to.'

'I know, but I thought I could control it.'

'Well, you clearly can't. Look at you, you're back where you was.'

'I know, I know. Please don't nag me.'

'You need more than a bleedin' good nagging! You promised Rachel that you'd never drink again. All those things you said to her, about how you regretted not raising her, how you wanted to make it up to her and be a good grandmother to Martha – did you mean any of it?'

'Of course I did!'

'Then prove it. Because believe me, Hilda, if you carry on like this, you'll lose them both forever and you'll end up in the gutter or dead. Is that what you want?'

'No.'

'Then you'd best pull your socks up.'

'Does Rachel know that I've been drinking?'

'No, not yet. But it won't be long before she finds out and then she'll be devastated. Surely you don't want to break her heart?'

'No, never.'

'Then stop bloody drinking! You can't have one or two glasses. You can't have any. Never.'

'I wish it was that easy, Win. What's the time? Eight, nine? And I'm already dying for a drink.'

'Have one, then. I'm not going to stop you. You're a grown woman, the choice is yours. But if you do, you can forget about ever seeing Rachel and Martha again. That's what it boils down to, Hilda. A whisky or your family?'

Winnie noticed Hilda's hands were shaking as she lit a cigarette. Though Hilda had said she'd only been drinking for a week, Winnie suspected it was worse than that.

'How do I stop drinking?'

'You have to make a decision and stick to it. It has to come from you. No one can do it for you. If you can't stop drinking for your daughter and your granddaughter, then nothing will stop you.'

'That's what scares me, Win.'

'You've done it before and you can do it again. This is just a hiccup.'

'Do you really believe I can?'

'Hilda, I *know* you can.'

Hilda poured her tea into her saucer and slurped a few mouthfuls. 'Thank you, Win. You're right. I can do it. And I've learned me lesson … I can't control the drink. The drink controls me. No more, not even a sniff. You won't tell Rachel, will you?'

'Not this time. But if you drink again, I won't hide the truth from her.'

'Thank you.'

'Drink your tea and get yourself cleaned up. Go and get your bath. I'll fill it up for you.'

'But it's freezin' in here.'

'It'll do you good. Go on, fetch your bath in.'

Hilda slowly stood up from the table and huffed. 'You can be a tough old boot sometimes, Win, but I don't know what I'd do without you.'

Hilda sloped away to the kitchen leaving Winnie feeling that she'd achieved what she'd set out to achieve. Now it was down to Hilda to prove that she could stay off the booze. And Winnie hoped with all her heart that Hilda would try, for all their sakes but especially for Rachel.

'Are you having trouble concentrating again, lad? Mr Beckett asked.

Bobby pulled his eyes away from gazing out of the shop window. 'Sorry. Yes, I am.'

'Your girl on your mind again?'

'Yes. I asked her to marry me.'

Mr Beckett chuckled as he turned the handle on the meat mincer. 'I remember the day that I asked my Doreen to marry me. I was a bag of nerves and before she could answer me, I dropped the ring. It rolled off the kerb and down a drain. We had a right fiasco retrieving it and it was covered in muck.'

'Look, here's the ring,' Bobby said enthusiastically. He pulled the small box from his trouser pocket and showed off the gold band with three small diamonds. The diamonds glinted brilliantly in the sunlight.

'What's that doing in your pocket? Shouldn't it be on Cheryl's finger?'

Bobby snapped the box shut. 'She hasn't said yes yet.'

'Yet?'

'She's thinking about it.'

'Well, it is a big decision to make.'

'Yes, and we've not been courting for long.'

'But she didn't say no.'

Bobby couldn't stop himself from smiling. 'What do you think she will say, Mr Beckett?'

'Don't ask me, lad. I've been married for over forty years and have three grown daughters but that doesn't mean I understand how a woman's mind works. They're mysterious creatures. But if she agrees to marry you, I can give you one bit of sound advice – never tell her that your mother is a better cook than her.'

Bobby was puzzled and asked, 'Why?'

'Goodness, lad, you've got a lot to learn,' Mr Beckett said. He tutted before chuckling again, and then went out to the back of the shop.

Bobby spent the rest of the day watching the minutes and hours tick by slowly. He was keen to get to see Cheryl and hoped she'd have an answer for him. When finally he arrived on her doorstep that evening, his heart was thumping hard.

He knocked on the door, clutching a small bunch of flowers. He hoped he'd be able to get a clue as to her decision from her face. She opened the door and smiled widely but Bobby still wasn't sure what her answer was going to be.

'Are they for me?' Cheryl asked.

'Yes.'

'Thank you. Come in, I'll put these in some water. Gran

346

is in the front room. She's looking forward to seeing you. She's got an article in the newspaper that she wants to show you about some strange meat that they eat in Africa. And be warned, she wants to know all the ins and outs about what you'll be doing with the Home Guard.'

After an hour or so, Bobby said that they should head down to the underground station. As they made their way down the hill, he whispered to Cheryl, 'Have you been thinking about what I asked you?'

She smiled. 'Yes, but I need to talk to my mum.'

'Your mum?' Bobby repeated in bewilderment. He would have thought that Mrs Hampton would be the last person that Cheryl would choose to discuss things with.

'Yes. Once I've spoken to my mum, I'll give you my answer. I promise.'

They trudged down the wooden-slatted escalator and through to the platform and their usual place. Bobby carried Edie's blankets as well as his own under one arm and had a bag with a flask, sandwiches and a pack of cards in the other. It wasn't heavy but he'd be pleased to unload and rest. But when they found their spot on the platform, he was disappointed to see that another family had taken it. Bobby sighed heavily. The platform was already filling up. They'd be hard pushed to find another area. He turned around to search for somewhere suitable but heard Cheryl's voice addressing the unwelcome family.

'That's our place,' she said abruptly.

'Got your name on it, has it?' the mother asked, equally sharply.

'No, but it's where we sleep every night.'

'You don't own it.'

'No, I don't, but it's *our* place.'

Bobby and the father looked at each other. It was clear that this was a problem for the women to sort out between them. After all, Bobby didn't care where they bedded down and it seemed that neither did the father. But he admired Cheryl's feistiness. That's my girl, he thought, proud of her.

'We was here first, so we ain't budging,' the mother said firmly.

'You bloody will, even if I have to drag you away!'

Edie cut in quickly, asking sweetly, 'Is it your first time down here, dear?'

'Yeah, but what of it?'

'Then you don't know that there's a protocol we all follow. You see, that's *our* place. You'll have to find somewhere else and then that will become *your* place. It's how it works. Don't go upsetting the apple cart, eh?'

The mother's face softened and she appeared to see reason. 'I'm sorry. We'll move.'

'Thank you.'

Bobby noticed that Cheryl's foot tapped impatiently as they waited for the family to gather their belongings. The small girl, probably about six or seven years old, let go of her older brother's hand and approached Cheryl. 'This is my dolly,' she said quietly. She held out a rag doll with dirty woollen hair.

Cheryl bent down and asked, 'What's her name? She's very pretty, just like you.'

'Her name is Wendy. She's my best friend.'

Bobby saw that the girl was little more than skin and bone, as was her brother. The family's clothes were old and worn and their blankets were almost threadbare. Cheryl must have

348

noticed too. She stood back up and asked the mother, 'Have you brought food and drinks with you?'

'We've got a bag of biscuits and a bottle of water.'

Cheryl looked at Bobby and indicated the shopping bag. 'Give them the sandwiches,' she whispered.

Bobby was touched by her kindness and rummaged in the bag. He handed Cheryl the wrapped sandwiches.

'Take these. We've all had our dinner. You can have my blankets too. It gets pretty cold down here.'

'Th-thank you. But I can't take your blankets,' the mother protested.

'Yes, have them. I can share with my gran.'

The mother gladly accepted the donations and the father shook Bobby's hand.

Bobby watched the poor family search for somewhere else to settle. The station was quickly filling, space was a premium. It was seven-thirty and the trains were still pulling in and out too.

'That was nice of you,' Edie said to Cheryl.

'That little girl, Gran. Did you see how hollow her eyes were?'

'Yes, poor mite. They all looked like they needed a good meal.'

'I don't understand,' Bobby chipped in. 'Everyone has ration coupons. I realise food is sparse, but we've all got enough to eat.'

'Maybe she isn't very good at managing her rations or maybe she has to exchange her coupons for other things.'

'Like what?'

'Perhaps she has to give them to the debt collectors. If

you can't pay your dues, they'll happily take your coupons,' Edie answered.

Bobby didn't know about that sort of thing. But he was pretty sure it was something that Errol would know about and wouldn't have been surprised if the bloke had taken family's ration books to clear debts owed him. Bobby had gathered from Cheryl that some of Errol's dealings had been pretty shady.

He saw the family leave the platform and assumed that they were heading to the other side. But he knew they'd find that platform just as full as this one.

A gush of wind forced its way through the tunnel. A train arrived but not many passengers disembarked. The train pulled away and then they heard the dreaded murmur travel along through the voices of the people sheltering in the station — the air-raid sirens had sounded. Bobby strained his ears to listen but couldn't hear the wailing. A crowd at the other end of the platform had begun to sing. Several children were crying. A train on the other platform rumbled into the station. The brakes screeched. There was the constant hum of nattering. All the sounds echoed in the tunnel and drowned out the noise from outside.

'Cup of tea?' Edie asked.

Bobby pulled the flask from the bag, grateful that Cheryl hadn't given that away too. 'Game of cards?' he asked.

'No, dear, you and Cheryl play. I'm going to do me knitting. I'm making a nice jumper for you for Christmas. Do you like the colour?'

Bobby did and he was touched by Edie's gesture. 'Thank you. Bottle-green is my favourite colour.'

He finished his small cup of tea and won the first two

hands of rummy with Cheryl. She pouted at him and he let her win the third.

'It's good of you to keep us company down here,' Edie said. 'Especially when you could be nice and comfy in the shelter in your garden.'

'I'd hardly call our shelter nice or comfy. Even if it was, I'd much rather be here with—' He stopped mid-sentence and caught his breath as a deafening boom filled the station. The cold ground of the platform beneath him shook and the place plunged into darkness. Men, women and children began to scream. Bobby felt a terror that he'd never known before and guessed that the ground above had been struck by a bomb. He sat, petrified, wondering what to do.

'What's happening?' Cheryl cried.

Her voice spurred Bobby into action. He jumped to his feet. He couldn't see Cheryl or Edie and reached through the pitch-blackness for them. 'Hold my hand,' he yelled.

He felt a hand in his. It was small and bony. Edie's. 'Cheryl – Cheryl – where are you?' he called.

'I'm here. Where's my gran?'

'Don't worry, I've got her. I'm right opposite you, Cheryl. Find my other hand.'

As Bobby fumbled in the darkness, he felt a wet and cold sensation begin to lap his feet. Water was coming from somewhere and it was flooding in fast. 'Cheryl, where are you? We've got to get out of here.'

'I'm here, Bobby. Go, go quickly. I'm right here.'

Bobby carefully stepped along the platform. He kept a firm grip of Edie's hand and kept calling for Cheryl.

'I'm with you. Keep going,' she answered.

The chilled water was now past his knees and he could

feel the force of it pushing against him as he waded through it. Other people in the dark jostled against him. He nearly lost his footing. As the water gushed in, panic was taking over all around. Everyone was fleeing for the exit but as they scrambled in the dark, the panic turned to mayhem.

'Argh,' Edie shrieked.

Bobby dared not let go of the old lady but he felt her tug away from him. Thankfully, he managed to keep a hold of her.

'I fell over,' she cried. 'I'm all right. Keep going.'

Bobby stumbled over something. He couldn't be sure but he feared he'd stepped on a body. And then another. 'Cheryl – Cheryl!'

He was so relieved when she shouted, 'I'm right behind you.'

The crowd was pushing him forward as he dragged Edie along. They managed to scramble over a pile of fallen debris. He fell, taking Edie with him. He felt an agonising pain as someone stepped on his free hand, crushing it against a brick beneath.

'Get up,' he screamed at Edie, 'Quickly, get up before we get trampled to death.'

'Go, Bobby. Leave me.'

'No. Come on, get up. We're nearly at the escalator.'

As Edie found her feet, over the sound of the cries and screaming, Bobby could hear the water rushing in. They climbed over the pile of debris and he found himself in waist-high water. He knew the escalators were just in front of them but so was a wall of people trying to escape. He found himself and Edie pushed up against them, being crushed by the people from behind. 'Cheryl – Cheryl!'

'I'm here,' she answered but her voice sounded further back.

The pressure of the people behind pressing against him felt terrifying. He could hardly breathe! Bobby began to climb the broken escalator. His foot went straight through the slatted step and he winced in pain as the wood splintered into his shin. But he managed to pull his leg free and to carry on up the stairs before anyone unwittingly shoved him to the ground and walked over him.

Edie was beginning to feel heavier. He knew she was struggling. But they had to get to the top. He felt another body underfoot and his stomach lurched.

'Cheryl – Cheryl!'

Her voice reached him but she sounded a long way down the escalator. 'Don't let go of my gran. Don't let go.'

Bobby wanted to turn around and run back to get her but he knew it was impossible. He was being forced to move forward and if he stopped, he and Edie would both be crushed.

'Can't breathe,' Edie groaned.

'Nearly there.' Bobby strained his eyes in the darkness. He could see the light from torches above. They were off the broken escalator and in the ticket hall. As people ran for the stairs which would take them to the street above, rescuers were coming down. The beam of a torch flashed across them. Bobby caught a glimpse of Edie. She looked bloodied and scared but she was alive, unlike so many on the escalator and platforms below.

He stood, staring back at the escalator, straining his eyes in the darkness, waiting for Cheryl to emerge. Several people barged into him. A continual flow of scared and screaming people rushed forward. Bobby pulled Edie to one side to avoid being knocked to the ground. Someone placed a hand on Bobby's shoulder. A warden.

'Come with me, Son. You're all right. And you, missus.'

'No – my girl—'

'My Cheryl,' Edie cried. 'We're waiting for Cheryl.'

'You can't wait here, it's not safe. You need to get upstairs.'

Reluctantly, Bobby allowed the man to lead them to the exit. He had to get Edie to safety. 'We're all right from here. Thank you,' he told the warden. As he walked up the steps, still gripping Edie's hand, people evacuating the station forced him forward. He became aware of the cold from his sodden clothes and he shivered. Edie was shivering too. He placed his arm over her trembling shoulders. 'I'll find her, Edie, I promise.'

'I know you will, but you can't go back down there.'

On the street, a woman from the voluntary service rushed towards them. She placed a blanket over Edie and ushered them towards a van. 'You'll get a hot drink here. Do you need to go to hospital?'

'No, I'm not going anywhere. My granddaughter is still down there.'

It was only now that Bobby could see the full extent of both their injuries. Blood trickled from Edie's eyebrow and her stockinged feet were bleeding. Bobby knew that his shin was badly cut and at least two of his fingers looked broken.

'She needs the hospital,' he told the woman. And then he said firmly to Edie, 'You must go. I won't leave here until I've found Cheryl and then we will both come straight to the Grove hospital for you.'

Edie nodded. She seemed to be dazed and allowed the woman to put her in the back of an ambulance. Bobby hobbled back towards the train station. He passed people sitting on the floor who were sobbing hysterically. The scene was horrific. There were several dead bodies around, a few with blankets covering their faces. Injured people were being carried from the ticket hall. A man was throwing up. A woman ran from left to right and then back again, calling her child's name. A young boy stood crying. He looked lost; his clothes were soaked through. But where was Cheryl? Bobby began to fear the worst. Was she still trapped down there? Trampled to death or drowned? She might have fallen through the broken escalator where his leg had slipped through. She could be crushed. No, not Cheryl. She was a fighter. He wouldn't allow himself to think that she could be dead.

Bobby ran against the emerging crowd of frightened people and back into the ticket hall. He scanned the area for Cheryl's face, calling her name and hoping to hear her sweet voice answer. Hundreds of scared and hurt people were coming towards him. Some, like him, were fighting against the throng to find their friends and family. A woman, her eyes blazing with fear that made her look insane, grabbed Bobby's arm. 'My baby – where's my baby?'

'I-I don't know,' Bobby stuttered.

She grabbed the next person, frantically asking the same question.

An old man collapsed in front of Bobby. He tried to help the man to his feet but was knocked over twice. The old man coughed and spluttered. His thin hair was dripping wet, as were his clothes. 'My wife,' he said breathlessly. 'She's still down there.'

Bobby managed to fight his way through the fleeing people

and he leaned the old man against a wall. 'Stay here. You're safe here,' he said.

He watched the swarm of men, women and children in the ticket hall all running for their lives. He thought that Cheryl had surely escaped by now. She hadn't been that far behind him. So many people had come up from the platforms. Cheryl *must* be amongst them somewhere and he must have missed her. He wandered back to the street and went from person to person looking for his love. He thought that she was probably looking for him and Edie too. He'd find her. He had to. The alternative was too painful to even imagine.

32

Cheryl's eyes slowly opened but everything was dark and she couldn't see anything. For a moment, she thought she'd gone blind. But then pain ripped through her body and she remembered. She'd been trying to escape from the underground station. She'd fallen over on the escalator and had been trampled. Fear engulfed her as she realised that she was trapped, buried under bodies.

The weight on top of her felt crushing. She couldn't move. She could feel the sharp edges of the escalator stairs underneath her, digging into her aching body. The muffled sound of whimpers and cries surrounded her. People were alive and trapped like her. She shook; her clothes drenched. But at least she was out of the flood.

Someone called for help. It was a woman's voice and she sounded close by. But Cheryl felt too weak to answer. She had to conserve what little strength she had left and prayed that someone would rescue her soon.

She tried to lift her head but she couldn't move. The person on top of her was too heavy. And then she was struck by a sickening thought – whoever was over her was dead!

She was lying trapped beneath a dead body. Cheryl squeezed her eyes shut. She wanted to scream. But she could hardly breathe, let alone screech.

The woman nearby called again for help. But no answer to her pleas came. Cheryl began to fear that no one was coming to save them. She thought she was going to die and when the rescuers finally arrived, they'd be digging out her corpse. She hoped that Bobby and her gran had escaped. The thought of her dear gran trapped like this sent a shudder through Cheryl.

Again, the woman cried out for help but her cry was met with silence.

Cheryl could feel her strength sapping away. *Must breathe*, she thought as she tried to draw in some air, but her chest could barely move. *Can't die ... must breathe.*

It felt helpless. There was nothing she could do to free herself. The excruciating agony in every part of her body was beginning to fade. Was this it? Was she dying? And then she heard another voice. A man's voice, one that she recognised. 'Reach out, Cheryl. Reach your hand out.'

'Dad?' she asked in the blackness. 'Dad – is that you?'

'Reach your hand out, Cheryl,' her father repeated.

'Where are you?'

'Reach out, my girl. Go on, sweetheart, you can do it.'

Cheryl, confused, did as her father instructed. She managed to push her hand up alongside a body beside her. She touched something. Another person? Another dead body?

Cheryl heard the woman who had been calling for help. 'Who's there? Who's touching me? Is someone there? Is anyone alive?' the woman asked.

Cheryl's fingers lightly tapped the woman.

'Oh, thank God. You're alive. I thought I was all alone down here. Can you speak?'

'I ... just,' Cheryl managed to croak.

'Hello? Are you still there? Can you hear me? Can you speak?'

The woman hadn't heard Cheryl's feeble reply so Cheryl tapped her again.

'Don't worry. I can talk. I'll keep shouting for help. I'll get us out of here.'

The woman's words were comforting but Cheryl didn't know for how much longer she could survive. The pain had numbed but now her body shook with the cold and her lungs ached for air.

'HELP US!' the woman yelled.

Cheryl had lost track of the length of time that they'd been trapped. She began slipping in and out of consciousness. When she was awake, she'd hear the woman continue to call for help but Cheryl noticed that the woman's voice was becoming hoarse and she sounded weaker too.

It felt as though she'd been buried alive for hours, possibly even days. She couldn't swallow. Breathing was almost impossible now. She passed out into blackness. Nothing. And when Cheryl woke again, her first thoughts were about Bobby. Her gran. Had she heard her dad's voice, or had she been dreaming? Her mum – she wished she'd made it up with her mum. She blacked out again.

'Help ... We're over here!' the woman called.

'It's all right, love, we've got you now.'

Cheryl's ears pricked. That was a man's voice! Someone had come to rescue them and not a moment too soon!

'Here … here … there's someone alive here – I felt them tapping me,' the woman said frantically.

Cheryl felt something warm in her free hand. It was another hand.

'Are you alive?' the man asked.

'Yes,' Cheryl answered but her voice was no more than a whisper.

'I think she's gone,' the man said.

'No – I'm alive,' Cheryl whispered. She squeezed the man's hand.

'Christ, she's alive! Quick, help me get her out.'

Cheryl didn't know what was going on above her but she felt the weight that had been crushing her finally lift and bright lights shone down on her, leaving her blinded.

'It's all right, miss, we'll get you out of here. You're going to be fine.'

Cheryl felt herself being lifted from the escalator and placed onto a stretcher. The pain began to flood back into her battered body. She groaned as she was carried into the ticket hall where she could now see the beautiful faces of the men who had saved her life. 'Thank you,' she said.

'What's your name, miss?'

'Cheryl Hampton. My boyfriend and my gran. They were with me. I don't know if they got out.'

'We need to get you to hospital.'

Cheryl's head slumped to the side. As she was taken through the ticket hall, she saw the aftermath of the disaster. Bodies laid everywhere. Thick dust hung in the air. She saw a man sitting crossed-legged on the ground. His head was hung low and he was rocking back and forth and crying. And then she noticed that he was holding a rag doll. A rag doll called Wendy. Tears fell from Cheryl's eyes and rolled into her bloodied hair. The man was the father of the little skinny girl that she'd met on the platform earlier and instinctively Cheryl knew that the child was dead.

As the men carrying her stretcher took her up the stairs to the street, the pain that wracked Cheryl's broken body became almost unbearable. 'It hurts,' she cried.

Outside, the air felt fresher. Cheryl closed her eyes against the sunlight. It had been evening when they'd gone down to the underground. She wondered how long she'd been down there. She opened her eyes again and looked from side to side, hoping to see Bobby or her gran. A row of waiting ambulances flanked the street. Fire engines too. So many people were standing and waiting to see who would be brought up from the station. Their worries were etched onto their faces.

As Cheryl was lifted into an ambulance, she glimpsed a view along the High Street. She thought her eyes were deceiving her. There, in the middle of the road, the rear end of a double decker bus stuck out from a huge crater in the ground. Glass blown out from shop windows littered the street and sparkled in the sunlight. People were standing around the hole in the ground and looking on in awe.

'Cheryl! Thank God, you're alive!'

Cheryl turned her head to see Bobby looking down at her. Relief washed over her. 'My gran,' she croaked.

'Edie is fine. She's at the hospital.'

He'd saved her gran. The man she loved had kept her gran alive.

'Yes,' Cheryl said, her voice barely more than a whisper. 'What?'

'My … answer … is yes.'

Before the ambulance doors were closed, Cheryl saw the biggest smile on Bobby's face and his eyes had welled with tears. *He's my fiancé*, she thought proudly. And she couldn't wait to tell her gran – and her mum.

33

Winnie woke on Tuesday morning with a feeling of gloom hanging over her. The local newspaper would be out today and she was dreading what had been printed about her, her family and her pub. In the kitchen, Rachel appeared chirpy and she told Winnie that she was silly to be worrying about it. But Winnie didn't want to be the target of the local gossips, especially as there were still some folk who gave her the cold shoulder. They blamed David for the motorbike accident that had left Brenda unable to walk. Winnie regretted now that she'd defended her son. He'd been wrong to walk away and leave Brenda lying injured in the street. And Winnie had been wrong to stick up for him.

'I'm taking Martha for a walk. Is there anything you want me to pick up while I'm out?' Rachel asked.

'No, thanks, love. I'll be going shopping myself later. But you could pop a letter to Jan into the post office for me. It's on the mantle in the other room.'

'Sure. I'll see you later.'

Once Rachel had left, Winnie wandered down to the pub. She stood with her hands resting on the bar as she looked

363

around. The place looked in good order, but she thought it was time for a change. Since Brian's death, the Battersea Tavern was solely hers. *Brian's death . . .* She'd hardly given her husband more than a second's thought. Instead, she'd poured out her grief over Harry. She wasn't even sure where Brian had been buried or who had buried him. Not that she cared. Winnie had very few fond memories of her husband and she had plenty of bad ones. Anyway, he was gone and would never be the bane of her life again. And now she wanted to rid the place of any semblance of him and give her pub a new look. It wouldn't be easy with a war on. She wasn't even sure if she'd be able to buy any paint. But at least she could start to make plans for the future.

Winnie checked the time. It was far too early to open. She wondered if the local paper had been delivered to the corner shop yet. She grabbed her coat off the newel post and hurried to the shop.

Len was coming out, his face grim.

'Morning, love. Everything all right?' she asked, concerned.

'Ain't you heard?'

'Heard what?'

'About Balham underground station.'

'What about it?'

'A bomb landed in the High Street. It broke the water mains and flooded the station. There was hundreds of people down there sheltering. Loads are dead, Winnie. They ain't said how many but they're still getting people out.'

Winnie's blood ran cold. 'Blimey, that's awful.'

'I know. Makes you think, don't it? Nowhere is safe.'

'I hope Harry's girl is all right. She's living in Balham with her gran.'

'Yeah, I hope so an' all. They reckon a lot of people drowned. The gates had been locked and the station master died with the keys on him. Must have been terrible for 'em.'

'I can't imagine, Len. Are you going home? I'll walk back with you.'

'Yeah, but I thought you was going to the shop?'

'I've changed my mind,' Winnie answered. The newspaper report suddenly seemed very unimportant.

Later that day, as her customers drifted in and out, the talk was mostly about the Balham underground disaster. Some people said that as many as three hundred souls had lost their lives. Others said twenty or thirty. There had been reports of gas leaks in the tunnels too. But whatever the truth was, the newspapers and wireless were playing down the horrendous incident. Winnie knew the full extent of the death toll was unreported in order to keep morale up. There were lots of things that the public were kept in the dark about. It was bad enough that they were weary from nightly raids, suffering food shortages and losing their sons and husbands on battlefields, let alone adding to the misery by banging on about the number of dead civilians in London. Winnie thought about Jan. She wondered if the injured from Balham had been taken to St Thomas's. *That girl deserves a medal for the work she's doing,* Winnie thought.

'Have you seen this?' Bernie asked. He placed a newspaper on the bar and pointed to a photograph of a bus sticking out of a big hole in the ground. 'It's where the bomb landed in Balham. The bus driver said he didn't see the hole, what with his dipped headlights and all that, and he drove straight into it.'

'He's lucky to be alive.'

'Cor, you can say that again.'

'Talking of newspapers, there's a story about you in the local rag.'

'So I believe.'

'Ain't you seen it?'

'No, and I've no desire to.'

'Can't say I blame you. They don't 'alf tell some fibs.'

Winnie's curiosity got the better of her and she asked, 'What sort of fibs?'

'Well, they said that you wouldn't allow any black-market trading in here, but we all know it was the place to come to see Harry.'

'Shush, will you,' Winnie hissed. 'I don't want to get in trouble with the law.'

'Oh, yeah, right, sorry, Winnie. But you should read it. The reporter has made you look like an angel.'

'Has he? I'm surprised. I wasn't exactly forthcoming with him.'

'You must have made a good impression on him. The same can't be said for Errol. He got slated, good job an' all.'

Winnie was pleased to hear that the newspaper had painted her in a kindly light. Not that it mattered. After what had happened in Balham last night, the local paper and its story about her seemed trivial.

When the door opened, Winnie looked past Bernie and was astonished to see Hilda walk in. Considering the woman was fighting to stay off the whisky, Winnie hadn't expected to see her in the pub for a while. Thankfully, Hilda was sober and she had cleaned herself up a treat.

'Hello, Win. All right if I go straight upstairs to see Rachel?'

'You don't have to ask, love. Martha will be glad of a

cuddle from her grandma. She's been a bit fretful. Teething, I think.'

Good, thought Winnie, pleased to see that Hilda was making a determined effort. It was such a shame that she had a drinking problem. If she hadn't, Winnie would have loved to offer Hilda the job of working in the pub and living upstairs. But she knew it could never happen. The temptation would be too much for Hilda and she'd likely lapse and end up drinking the place dry.

'You're awake,' Edie said with delight.

'Am I in hospital, Gran?' Cheryl asked groggily.

'Yes, dear. And you will be for a while. You've got several broken ribs, a broken arm and ankle and you've had stitches in your legs, head and shoulder. But you're alive and you'll mend.'

'How are you?' Cheryl asked. She was trying to put on a brave face and not let on to her gran about how much pain she was in.

'Just a few cuts and bruises. Bobby's fine too, a couple of broken fingers and stitches in his leg. He's a good lad; he got me out of there. If it wasn't for him, well, I dread to think.'

Cheryl tried to smile but everything hurt. Memories flooded into her mind of being pinned down on the escalator by a dead body. And the rag doll. How many people had been killed?

Her gran smoothed back a loose piece of hair from Cheryl's brow. 'You look exhausted. Rest, dear. I'll be sitting right here. I shan't let you out of my sight again,' she said reassuringly.

Cheryl closed her eyes, but when she did, an overwhelming feeling of panic made her heart race. She felt as though she was back in the station, alone in the darkness and fighting for her life.

'I can't sleep,' she cried. Tears slipped from her eyes and Edie wiped them away gently.

'It's all right, dear. Just lie there quietly instead.'

'It was horrid. I thought I was going to die.'

'I know. But you didn't. You can't allow yourself to think about that.'

'The little girl, the one with the rag doll – she's dead, Gran.'

'Shush, now. You're getting yourself all worked up. Bobby will be here soon. You don't want him seeing you like this, do you?'

'I can't help it. I'll never forget how I felt and what I saw.'

'None of us will. But we can't dwell on it. Look, you've started me off now,' Edie said, dabbing at her tears.

'Oh, Gran, please don't cry. I'm sorry.'

'I'll stop if you stop.'

Cheryl managed a weak smile.

'That's better. You've a beautiful smile, Cheryl.'

Cheryl looked away, knowing that there was a deep sadness behind her smile. Even Bobby's cheerful voice did nothing to lift the gloom that engulfed her.

'Hello, my love. How are you feeling?'

'Miserable,' Edie answered for her.

'Well, she's been through a lot. And I should imagine she's in a lot of pain.'

'I'll say. The poor girl must be very sore.'

As her gran and Bobby discussed her health, Cheryl's mind drifted back to the escalator again. Her dad had saved her life. He'd told her to reach out. If she hadn't put her hand

368

out, she might not have been rescued alive. It couldn't have been a dream. His voice had been so clear. 'Do you believe in ghosts?' she asked.

Her gran and Bobby looked at each other bewildered and then back at her.

'Why do you want to know?' Edie asked.

'My dad was with me – on the escalator. He told me what to do to save my life.'

'You heard him?' Bobby asked.

'Yes, as clear as day.'

'Did you see him?' her gran asked.

'No, I couldn't see anything, it was too dark. But I heard him. I know it was my dad.' Cheryl looked at both their faces and knew that neither of them believed her. But that didn't matter. She knew the truth. Her dad had looked after her. She wondered if he was with her now. Was he sitting on the edge of her bed? If only she could hear him again.

'Perhaps it was someone else down there with you who sounded like your dad,' her gran suggested.

'No, it was him.'

'Well, I'm glad he was with you. I feel terrible about leaving you alone down there,' Bobby said.

'It wasn't your fault, Bobby. I'm so grateful that you was with my gran.'

'All the same, I'll never leave you again. Have you told your gran?'

'Told me what?' Edie asked.

Cheryl quickly shook her head as she remembered that she'd agreed to marry him. But she'd been wrapped up in the moment when she'd said 'yes'. Now, with a sore head and aching body, marriage was the last thing on her mind and she still wanted to discuss it with her mother.

'Well, is one of you going to tell me?' Edie pushed.

'I asked Cheryl to marry me and she said yes!'

Edie clapped her hands together with delight. 'Oh, that's wonderful news. I'm so happy for you both. You make a lovely couple.'

'Thanks, Edie. I'm over the moon.'

'Call me Gran,' Edie said. 'Will you be moving in with us after the wedding?'

'I don't know; we haven't talked about anything yet.'

Bobby was full of enthusiasm but Cheryl looked away. Her thoughts were still in the underground station and she wanted her mum more than ever. She couldn't bring herself to tell Bobby that she still wasn't sure about getting married, especially as he sounded so happy.

'You look worn out,' Bobby said gently. 'I think we should go and leave you to rest.'

Cheryl slowly moved her head back round to look at him. She burst into tears and an anguished cry left her lips as she sobbed uncontrollably. 'Please don't leave me,' she cried.

Bobby leaned over her but due to her injuries, he was unable to hold her.

'It's all right, my love. We won't leave you.'

Cheryl cried her eyes out until she had no more tears left. 'I'm sorry,' she muttered, breathless. It hurt to inhale. Her head was pounding. Everything was sore and she felt sick. She knew her body would repair and eventually it would feel better but she doubted that her mind would ever get over the horrors of being trapped in the station.

Bobby gently stroked the back of her hand. 'I should have

been with you. But when you're hurting like this, remember that your dad was with you. Take comfort in knowing that you wasn't alone.'

'Thank you. You're right. I'll try and remember that.'

'That's my girl.'

'Do you feel a bit better now?' Edie asked.

'Yes, I think I do. But I'm so tired,' she answered. She didn't admit to either of them that she needed her mum beside her. They wouldn't understand.

'Close your eyes and think about your wedding day. Imagine the dress that you'll wear. Your flowers. How you'll have your hair styled. We'll be sitting right here with you.'

'Thanks, Gran,' Cheryl whispered. She closed her eyes and hoped she wouldn't see the rag doll again or feel the fear of thinking that she was taking her last breathes. *My dress*, she thought. *Think about my dress.* Cheryl wasn't even sure that she wanted to be married just yet and she'd always imagined that when she did tie the knot, her mum would help her choose her dress. She had hoped it would have brought them closer. All she ever wanted was a relationship with her mother like Yvonne had with hers. A sad thought crossed Cheryl's mind: had her mum ever loved her? She'd never been shown any affection. Cheryl hated herself for craving it. She wished that she didn't feel that she needed her mum so much. But, at least she could take solace in knowing that her dad had loved her and she was sure of that. She'd always remember his voice telling her to reach out. As the darkness engulfed her, the fear returned and Cheryl fell into a fretful sleep, reliving the underground station tragedy in her nightmares.

34

The following day, once the pub had closed after lunchtime, Winnie pulled her coat on, wrapped her scarf over her head and then called up the stairs, 'I'm off out shopping. See you later.'

'See you,' Rachel called back.

Winnie grabbed her shopping basket from behind the counter and set off for the greengrocer's. As she trudged along the street, she made a mental note of what she needed. Spuds, carrots, parsnips, maybe a turnip. If she could get her hands on a bit of mutton, she could make a nice pot of stew that would last them for a couple of days.

As Winnie joined the queue in the grocer's, her mind was on Christmas. But then her thoughts were interrupted when she heard a familiar voice in front of her, at the counter. It was Carmen and, to Winnie's astonishment, the woman was begging the grocer.

'Just a couple of spuds, please. You've known me for years and I've always been a good customer.'

'I'm sorry, Mrs Hampton, but if you've got no money, then you can't have any veg.'

'Thanks for nothing,' Carmen spat. She spun on her heel and marched out of the shop.

Winnie stared after the woman in disbelief. Carmen was down on her luck but Winnie had been appalled to hear her begging for a couple of potatoes. She was tempted to ignore Carmen's hardship and to let the horrible cow get on with it, but, against her better judgement, she dashed out of the shop and chased after her.

She found Carmen sitting on the step outside the café. The woman looked downbeat and, though Winnie didn't like her, she couldn't help but feel sorry for her. She wondered if Carmen had heard about the bomb and fatalities in Balham. No woman, no matter how horrid a character, should ever have to worry about the death of her daughter. Winnie knew what that felt like. It hadn't been that long ago when she'd been standing by a pile of debris and waiting to hear if Jan had been killed. But the look on Carmen's face told Winnie that the woman was oblivious to the events in Balham. 'Hello, Carmen,' she said casually.

Carmen glared up from the step with angry eyes. 'Come to gloat, have you?'

'No, not at all. I've come to see if you're all right?'

'No, of course I bleedin' ain't! My husband is dead and my son has been locked up and me daughter doesn't want to know me. I've been left with nothing. Nothing. There, now you know. Now you can go and stand behind your bar and tell everyone how the stuck-up Carmen Hampton has been reduced to begging for something to eat. You can all have a laugh and it'll give 'em something to talk about.'

Carmen's outburst had been expected. But Winnie was

undeterred. 'Come inside, eh? We can have a cuppa. It's cold out here.'

'Are you paying?'

Winnie nodded.

'I ain't too proud to turn down a cuppa.'

They sat at a window table in the corner and when the waitress came over, Winnie ordered two cups of tea and sandwiches for them both.

'I never thought I'd be accepting charity from you again.'

'It's not charity, Carmen. There's a war on, we all have to help each other out.'

'Call it what you want, it's still charity in my eyes.'

When their tea and food was served, Carmen ate hungrily. Winnie could only manage half her own sandwich and she pushed her plate across the table to Carmen. Their eyes met and Winnie was sure she saw a spark of gratitude in Carmen's.

Carmen finished her food and sipped her tea. 'I suppose you're wondering how I ended up in this state?'

'It's none of my business.'

'That don't wash with me, Winnie. I bet you're dying to know.'

'No, not really.'

'What's the matter? Don't you want to hear your precious Harry being bad-mouthed?'

'No, and he was never *my* precious Harry.'

'No he weren't, and you should thank your lucky stars that he weren't. It was me who was lumbered with him and look how he's left me!'

'What do you mean?'

'I'm skint, Winnie. I don't have a pot to piss in, thanks to him.'

'It wasn't Harry's fault that your house got destroyed.'

'You don't know the half of it. You think Harry was this great bloke who made everyone laugh and was such a wonderful husband and father. Well, it weren't like that. He was useless.'

'You shouldn't speak ill of the dead, Carmen.'

'I'll speak how I like about him. I had to put up with him for most of my life and look where that got me.'

'He was a loyal husband, Carmen. Regardless of what you think, nothing ever went on with me and him.'

Carmen smiled sardonically. 'Harry didn't know the meaning of loyal. I should have let you have him. You would soon have found out for yourself what a waste of space he was.'

Winnie looked down into her cup of tea. She couldn't stand to hear Carmen saying mean things about Harry and it was all she could do to restrain herself from lashing out at the woman. She was beginning to think that it had been a bad idea to have offered a helping hand to Carmen. She was about to scrape her chair back and march out of the café but Carmen continued talking.

'You're a sensible woman, Winnie. You run your own business and from what I saw, very well too. But Harry would have bled you dry. Money went through his hands like water. Easy come, easy go. That was him. The man had no sense of responsibility and couldn't see past the end of his nose. He lived for the moment, not caring about the next day or where the money was going to come from to put food on the table.'

'You and yours always had the best of everything. You didn't do badly with Harry.'

'Yes, thanks to me! I've spent my life squirrelling money away from him so that he didn't blow it on flash clothes

375

and fancy things for the home. He was a spendthrift. I had to badger him for the housekeeping and put away what I could or he'd blow it all. The amount of money that came through that house, we could have bought it fifty times over but oh no, Harry had to buy everyone in the pub a drink to make sure he was popular. Or he'd go out and buy Cheryl an expensive dress and Errol a suit, buying their love. Woe betide he'd ever discipline the pair of them. No, that was left down to me so that I always looked like the mean parent.'

'That doesn't make him a bad person. Just generous to a fault.'

'Really? Is that what you think? Let me tell you where most of his money went, then see how generous you think he was – prostitutes. He spent a fortune on visiting them. In fact, he spent more on whores than he ever did on me. I always knew when he'd seen one of his tarts because he'd come home reeking of cheap perfume and bringing me a gift to ease his guilt.'

Winnie gaped, open-mouthed, at Carmen. Surely the woman was mistaken or telling lies?

'I can see you're shocked. Sweet Harry with whores. But it's true. It started when I was carrying Cheryl and refused to meet his "needs". He took his pleasure elsewhere. It suited me at the time but he carried on seeing them after Cheryl was born. Two, three, sometimes four times a week. And you know Harry, he had expensive tastes. Only the best would do for him. The tarts didn't come cheaply.'

Winnie was gobsmacked.

'I asked him to stop but he wouldn't. He insisted it meant nothing and that he loved me. When he gave me a disease, I couldn't have him in my bed after that. But I couldn't throw him out either. He was the provider, for what it was worth.'

The waitress cleared their plates and Winnie asked for another two cups of tea. She was beginning to see Harry in a most unfavourable light. 'That must have been horrible for you,' she said, finding herself at a loss for words.

'Yes, it was. I know what everyone thinks of me. You all reckon I'm a bitch and a stuck-up cow. But I'm not. Harry made me what I am – a bitter woman, ashamed of her life. He humiliated me so I distanced myself from our friends and neighbours and hoped that the truth about what he got up to would never come out. It was bad enough when I had to get treated by the doctor. I thought I'd die of shame. Honestly, Winnie, it was one of the worst experiences of my life.'

'I can imagine!'

'And I was worried for Cheryl too. She would have been shattered if she'd known about her father's "interests". She idolised the man, more fool her. But I didn't want to see the girl upset.'

'You put up with a lot.'

'I did. I should have left him years ago but I never had the nerve. I kept quiet and got on with it. We do though, don't we?'

Winnie thought about the years she'd tolerated Brian's abuse. 'Yeah, we do.'

'And to tell you the truth, I was worried that if I said anything about it, then he'd spurt out about my past – I'm a bastard. My mother had a one-night fling with a gypsy and nine months later, out I popped.'

Winnie thought of Alma, the baby she'd given up for adoption against her will, and Martha, her granddaughter, born to an unmarried mother. 'That's nothing to be ashamed of,' she said.

'You know how people talk and what they say.'

'Take no notice. It's just ignorance. Look at my Martha – you couldn't find a bonnier girl and Rachel is such a good mother.'

Carmen rubbed her finger on her forehead, her eyes squeezed shut. When she opened them again, she looked Winnie directly in the eyes. 'I've said wicked things about Rachel. And about you. When really, if I'm honest, it was myself and my life that I hated. I feel terrible about the poison that's come out of my mouth. Bitterness changes a person, Winnie. I don't want to be like that anymore. I should take a leaf out of your book and try being kinder.'

'You ain't got a pot to piss in but kindness costs nothing,' Winnie said. She was finding herself warming to Carmen. Behind her hard exterior, she was a good woman who'd been dealt a rough hand. She appreciated Carmen's honesty and remembered the *old* Carmen, whom she'd first met over twenty years ago.

'You're right there. I'm absolutely bleedin' brassic. Harry never did an honest day's work in his life. I can't get any help from the Government. Errol was looking after me but now he's got himself locked up so I'm going to be thrown out of my house. I don't know what to do ...'

Winnie was horrified when Carmen began to cry. The woman's defences were down and she'd shown her vulnerability and sadness.

'Sorry,' Carmen snivelled. 'It's not your problem. After all my savings went up in smoke with my house, and that useless husband of mine hardly brought home a penny before he died. I've nothing put by. Not a bean.'

Winnie suddenly realised that her suspicions about Errol had been correct. He hadn't been working with his father but against him. 'Did you know that Errol had taken over Harry's business?'

Carmen shot Winnie an incredulous look.

'It's true. He was selling in my pub. I assumed he was working with Harry but now I can see what really went on.'

'The bastard,' Carmen hissed. 'My own flesh and blood would oust my husband and leave us skint. That explains why we had no money coming in. I can't believe Errol would have done such a thing. Well, stuff him. He can rot in prison, for all I care. I heard what he did to you; I'm really sorry. I'm ashamed of him. I thought I raised him better than that. He should have known that it's never all right to hit a woman.'

'It's not your fault, love. There's no need for you to apologise for what he did to me. I don't blame you or Harry. I know you raised him well.'

Carmen then divulged another secret. 'Harry wasn't his father,' she said.

This didn't come as much of a surprise to Winnie. 'I guessed that,' she said. 'Errol made a point of saying that Harry wasn't his dad.' She didn't mention that Harry had told her too.

'Errol's father was Harry's brother, Wilf. I was going to marry Wilf but Harry charmed me away and I ended up with the wrong brother. I've lived my life regretting that decision.'

'We all make mistakes when we're young – and when we're old too.'

'Harry's mother tried to stop our wedding. I wish she

had done. She would have saved me from a lifetime of grief. Cheryl's living with her now and she's not speaking to me. Again, thanks to Harry.'

'Why?'

'We told the kids that their gran was dead. They grew up not knowing her. Me and Edie never got on; she looked down her nose at me, but I wouldn't have denied her the right to see her grandchildren. It was Harry. He didn't want her in our lives. See, Wilf was always her favourite and she made no secret of it. Harry was made to feel that he wasn't good enough compared to his brother. He held a lot of resentment. But to be fair, Wilf was a nicer bloke than Harry. Edie always used to go on about how wonderful Wilf was and she'd pick out all of Harry's faults. She was a strong woman and Harry was weak. Rather than front her, he cut her out of his life and persuaded me to do the same. He said he didn't want her belittling him in front of the kids. And then, over the years, I suppose it suited me too because I knew that Edie never believed that Errol was Harry's son. I was scared that she'd say something about it.'

Winnie understood all too well what it was like to harbour secrets. She'd kept Alma a secret for years and had held Brian's vile secrets too. But she'd learned that they always came out in the end. Just as Carmen's secrets had. 'These things have a way of coming back to bite you on the bum.'

'Cor, don't they! I hope I can make it up with Cheryl, but I'm hardly in a position to try right now. I need to sort myself out first. I don't want her feeling sorry for me. But now she's got Edie, she might not want anything more to do with me and, to be honest, I can't blame the girl.'

Winnie looked down into her lap and wondered if she

should tell Carmen about Balham tube station. Maybe Edie had an Anderson in her back garden and Cheryl had been safe in that. But maybe not. 'I'm sorry to tell you this, but there's been a terrible accident in Balham.'

'What sort of accident?' Carmen asked, frowning.

'A bomb landed on the High Street near the underground. It burst a water mains pipe and flooded the station. Hundreds of people were down there sheltering. Do you know if Edie has a shelter in her garden?'

'I've no idea. Oh, God, Cheryl might have been down there! What do I do, Winnie? Oh my God, what do I do?'

'It's all right. Calm down. Cheryl is probably safe and well. Try not to worry. I'll help you find out.'

'How? How can we find out?'

'Do you know where Edie lives?'

Carmen nodded furiously. 'But I don't have the bus fare or anything.'

'Don't worry about that. Come on, we'll get a taxicab straight there.'

Winnie rushed over to the counter and paid the bill. She glanced over her shoulder to Carmen. The woman was wringing her hands and was clearly shaken.

Thankfully, they soon found a taxicab and after a fraught half-hour later, Winnie stood back as Carmen hammered on Edie's front door.

'There's no answer,' Carmen said frantically and she knocked again.

The next-door neighbour came out and asked if she could help.

'I'm looking for Edie and my daughter, Cheryl. Do you know if they were in the tube station?'

The woman cleared her throat before answering. 'Yes, they were. We were too. It was pandemonium. I'm sorry; I can't tell you if they got out or not.'

'How can I find out?'

'I don't know. Sorry.'

'Come on,' Winnie said with authority. 'We'll go down to the station.'

Winnie struggled to keep up with Carmen, who was almost running down the hill. As they approached the station, Winnie was shocked at what she saw and her heart sank. Carmen ran on ahead and was talking to a warden. When Winnie caught up with her, Carmen was frantic.

'She's not on his list. She could be at the hospital. The Grove.'

'Right, let's get over there.'

After another tense drive in a taxicab to Tooting, they were outside the hospital. Carmen was out of the taxi like a hare out of a trap and she rushed into the building. Winnie paid the fare and found Carmen looking anxious but with a smile on her face.

'She's alive, Winnie. She's on a ward.'

'Come on, then, let's go and see her.'

'I-I don't know. What shall I say to her? She won't want to see me.'

'I'm sure she'll want to see you. Just pop in and say hello. Ask her how she is. Tell her that you're sorry and how much you love her.'

'I don't think I can. I've never said anything like that to her before.'

'Then now is the time. I'll wait here for you.'

'No, I'd rather you came with me – if you don't mind?'

Outside the ward, Winnie had to almost push Carmen through the doors. A nurse directed them to a bed and told them that they couldn't stay long as Miss Hampton already had visitors and needed to rest.

'I bet Edie is with her,' Carmen whispered. 'This is going to be awkward.'

Winnie recognised the old woman sitting by Cheryl's bed – and the bloke beside her. She couldn't remember his name, was it Robby? Something like that. When Edie spotted Carmen, she glared fiercely at her and jumped from her seat.

'What are you doing here?' Edie hissed.

'I'm here to see my daughter.'

'She doesn't want to see you, so bugger off!'

'No. Not before I've said me piece.'

'We don't want to hear anything you have to say.'

Winnie wasn't sure if she should interfere or not but gently she said, 'Please, Edie, let Carmen speak.'

'Huh, you've changed your tune. Have you forgotten what happened in your pub?'

'No, but I've had a good chat with Carmen and, well, I think you should let Carmen explain.'

'Please, I want to see my mum,' Cheryl said, her voice weak.

Edie's eyebrows rose in surprise at Cheryl's words but she said, 'Go on, then, let's hear it. But you'd better not upset her.' Edie stood to one side and allowed Carmen closer to the bed.

Winnie saw that Cheryl had been badly injured but she was conscious and looking at her mother, though Winnie couldn't gauge if Cheryl was pleased to see her or not.

'Hello, Cheryl,' Carmen said softly. She smiled awkwardly

at her daughter and Winnie could sense how uncomfortable Carmen felt.

When Cheryl responded with a curt, 'Hello', Winnie silently urged Carmen to continue.

'Is that it?' Edie asked. 'Have you only come to say hello?'

Carmen shook her head. Winnie knew that the woman was struggling to find the words. *Just say it*, Winnie thought. *Say you're sorry*.

Edie spoke again. 'She's hurt and she's tired. You've seen that she's alive so you might as well bugger off now.'

At last, Carmen found her voice. 'I'm sorry. I'm sorry to both of you,' she said, and then she glanced over her shoulder at Edie, who looked unimpressed. 'I did a lot of things wrong. I've made a lot of mistakes. I'm sorry for all of it. I don't want to lose you, Cheryl. You're my daughter and ... and ...' Her voice trailed off.

Say it, Winnie urged again in her head.

Carmen sucked in a large lungful of air and then spoke loudly and clearly. 'And I love you.'

Winnie saw a tear trickle from Cheryl's eye.

'I hope you can forgive me, you and Edie.'

Edie sniffed but her face softened. 'I won't be around forever; she'll need her mother. I'll never like you, Carmen, but I can put up with you for Cheryl's sake. If that's what she wants?'

There was a long, tense silence while they waited to see how Cheryl would respond. Winnie crossed her fingers and hoped that some sort of happy ending would come from this.

'Say it again,' Cheryl croaked.

'I'm sorry,' Carmen repeated.

'No, not that.'

Carmen looked around at Winnie and smiled. Then she turned back to Cheryl and said proudly, 'I love you.'

Cheryl smiled too and with tears in her eyes, she muttered, 'I'm getting married, Mum. What do you think of that?'

'Oh, oh, that's lovely. Congratulations. You must be the lucky man?' Carmen gushed, turning to Robby or whatever his name was.

'Yes, I'm Bobby,' he answered.

Carmen looked delighted. Her dark eyes glistened with tears of happiness. Cheryl was beaming and crying too. The scene brought a tear to Winnie's eye as well.

The nurse came by and reminded them that their visiting time was over. Edie discreetly explained to Carmen how afraid Cheryl was of being left alone and, given the horrific circumstances of what had happened to her, the hospital had permitted Bobby to stay. 'But I'm going home today, so I suppose I should invite you back to my house for a cuppa?' Edie's offer was said with a notable amount of disdain.

'Thank you,' Carmen replied politely. 'But you should probably get some rest too. I'd like that, though, one day, when you're feeling up to it.'

'Hmm,' Edie answered and she looked at Carmen as though she were dog's muck on the bottom of her shoe.

It was obvious that Edie and Carmen were never going to be the best of friends but at least the women were tolerating each other.

'Can we offer you a lift home?' Winnie asked.

'Have you got a motorcar?'

'No, we came in a taxicab.'

'I see. Thanks, but they're very expensive. I'm quite happy on the bus.'

'I'd rather we dropped you home.'

Edie looked sideways at Carmen. Winnie knew the old woman didn't want to spend a minute longer with Carmen than she had to.

'I'll get the bus, but thanks all the same.'

Winnie thought the woman must be as strong as an ox or just plain stubborn. Edie looked worn out and was injured too. In fact, Winnie was surprised that the hospital was even allowing her home. But she supposed they must need the beds for those who were more seriously hurt.

'You don't have to speak to me in the taxicab and I won't speak to you,' Carmen offered.

'In that case, I'll be glad to be dropped home,' Edie said. 'These shoes aren't mine. I lost mine in the station. These are far too big for me. I'm not sure I can walk far in them.'

The journey to Edie's house was made in silence, the old woman only speaking to thank Winnie as she climbed out of the taxicab.

'The Battersea Tavern, please,' Winnie instructed the driver. 'You did well today,' she told Carmen.

Carmen nodded but seemed deep in thought and Winnie could guess what was on her mind. 'Are you worrying about what you're going to do next?' she asked.

'Yeah. Without Errol to pay my rent, I'm going to be homeless.'

Winnie patted the back of Carmen's hand, her mind turning. As they drove to Battersea, she hardly noticed the bomb sites or the children carrying gas masks. The long queues outside the shops, the soldiers or the government posters everywhere.

They arrived outside the pub and Winnie told the driver to wait a moment while she dashed inside to get some money.

'Will you stay with him? I won't be a tick,' she asked Carmen.

Inside, Rachel was just coming down the stairs. 'I was getting worried about you, you've been gone ages,' she said.

'Sorry. Listen, I've got to be quick, I've got a taxicab outside.'

'What's going on?' Rachel asked.

Winnie briefly explained and then went back outside and paid the driver.

'Thank you for everything,' Carmen said. 'I'll pay you back one day, when I can.'

'No need. You can work it off.'

'What do you mean?'

'There's plenty of shifts going begging behind my bar.'

'Are you offering me a job?'

'Yes.'

'Why on earth would you want to do that?' Carmen asked suspiciously.

'Because I can.' Winnie hoped she wouldn't regret this and blurted, 'Come and live in the pub and work behind the bar with me. I need someone I can trust.'

Carmen's eyebrows rose and she stared at Winnie, her mouth agape.

'But you'd have to be nice to my customers and not scare 'em off,' Winnie added and she chuckled.

'You'd offer me a home and a job? After the way I've spoken to you in the past?'

'I know, I must need me head testing, but yes, why not?

You need a job and I need a barmaid. I've had a quick word with Rachel and she doesn't object.'

'I'm not sure ...'

'Why? Have you got a better offer?'

'No, but—'

'The past is behind us. We're both widows who were married to men who treated us badly. Let's write a new future for us, eh? A good one. We deserve it.'

A smile slowly spread across Carmen's face. 'I don't know what to say ...'

'"Yes" would be a good start.'

'Yes! Thank you, Winnie, you've saved my life!'

'I wouldn't go as far as to say that,' Winnie said. 'Go and pack. You're moving in with us.'

Who'd have thought it! Never in a million years would Winnie have believed that she and Carmen would even be on speaking terms. But now that Carmen had dropped her 'hard cow' act and showed more of her softer side, Winnie thought they could all rub along together quite nicely. They had a lot in common and she hoped that Carmen would soon become a valued asset to the Battersea Tavern and a good friend too.

As Carmen went off to pack, Winnie hoped that she'd made the right decision. Only time would tell. But how much time? With frequent bombing raids, the future was uncertain. The Battersea Tavern was her home, her granddaughter's home and her business too. Inwardly she prayed that it would remain standing. For as long as it did, she'd be there, behind the bar with a smile of welcome on her face for her customers.

Winnie stiffened her shoulders with resolve as she walked back into her pub and hoped this stinking war would end soon. Surely it would. And then the children could return to London from the countryside. And the fighting, battle-weary men could come home to their wives and mothers. Terry and Jan could marry. Now that was something to look forward to! And, who knew, maybe even Rachel would find herself a nice fella. But in the meantime, as they buried loved ones and cleaned up the destruction from Hitler's bombs, Winnie was ready to pour a pint and offer tea and sympathy where needed. The Battersea Tavern was at the heart of the community and, though Winnie didn't know it, she was in the hearts of all those who frequented her fine establishment.

Acknowledgements

I'd like to say a big thank you to Tracy Robinson, Beverley Ann Hopper, Sandra Blower and Lucy Gibbo Gibson for running the smashing Kitty Neale and Sam Michaels Fan Group. We lost a dear friend, but Jay Angel Griffin will always have a place in our hearts.

I'd also like to thank my wonderful editor, Francesca Pathak. You are an absolute joy to work with, and so are the rest of the fabulous team at Orion!

And it goes without saying that I'd like to thank all my readers for your continued support.

Lastly, but not least, Deryl Easton. Thank you for sharing your inspiring family stories with me xxx

Credits

Kitty Neale and Orion Fiction would like to thank everyone at Orion who worked on the publication of *A Family Secret* in the UK.

Editorial
Francesca Pathak
Lucy Brem

Copy editor
Marian Reid

Proof reader
Kati Nicholl

Audio
Paul Stark
Jake Alderson

Contracts
Anne Goddard
Ellie Bowker
Humayra Ahmed

Design
Rachael Lancaster
Joanna Ridley
Nick May
Helen Ewing

Editorial Management
Charlie Panayiotou
Jane Hughes
Tamara Morriss

Finance
Jasdip Nandra
Afeera Ahmed
Elizabeth Beaumont
Sue Baker

Marketing
Brittany Sankey

Discover how Winnie's story began with the heartwrenching first book in the Battersea Tavern saga

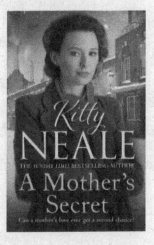

Can she put right the secrets of the past?

London, 1939. Winnie Berry has been the landlady of the Battersea Tavern for nearly twenty-five years, and the pub is like home to her – a place of tears and laughter, full of customers that feel like family. A place where she's learned to avoid the quick fists of her husband, and where she's raised her beloved son, David.

He's inherited his father's lazy streak and can't seem to hold down a job, but when war is declared Winnie is determined to keep her son safe. She's still haunted by the choice she made years ago as a desperate young woman, and she won't make the same mistake of letting her family be taken from her...

But when a young woman crosses her path, the secrets of Winnie's past threaten to turn her world upside down. There's nothing stronger than a mother's love – but can it ever have a second chance?